Chris Maxwell has a brain infection and his success explanation.

My perspective of Chris Maxwell has evolved from that of a casual acquaintance in our youth to a valued personal friend with whom I share a weekly morning breakfast and intimate life conversations. In Chris' youth, long before his illness shattered life as he knew it, Chris was the epitome of a flamboyant extrovert with a dynamic personality and unbridled energy. Chris now leads a very busy life of counseling, speaking engagements, travel, teaching, and authoring numerous books. He does so in a quite measured, incremental, intentional, and methodical manner. His mastery of technology and adaptation to somewhat rigid, self-enforced personal habits and schedules contribute to his success. His management of his residual brain disorders and their daily challenges go unnoticed by most folks. If Chris didn't share his story, I'm certain most people would be unaware of the "valley of death" which once threatened to destroy his brain and swallow his life, and they would also be in awe of the height of the mountaintops he subsequently climbed!

As a physician, I understand the medical ramifications of Chris Maxwell's near-death brain infection and its resulting brain insult. As his friend, it is remarkable to witness Chris' ability to turn his nightmarish medical crisis and disability into a source of inspiration, encouragement, and hope for others. He endeavors to tell his story for the benefit of humanity.

Chris Maxwell's story brings new dimension, deeper insight, and refreshing perspective. I am pleased he has chosen to share it!

– James R. Swails, M.D.

I was hired on pastoral staff after Chris had returned to work. I never knew Chris before his illness but realized quickly that he had become a new man. People would recount stories of the former Chris with great pride and a sense of community. Even with the difficulties of names, recollection of facts and dates, and the visual discomfort it caused Chris, people continued to crave his investment in their lives. He was still their pastor.

Chris mourned his prior self, was frustrated at his limitations, longed to work all day without naps, and wept at the pain that his family had suffered. Yet in all of this, I witnessed a man who grew and accomplished greatness. Chris worked extremely hard to overcome and would constantly strive to improve. There were many days when Chris pushed too hard and would have to stop and regroup. These setbacks would become fuel to move forward. Chris would comment daily on his small victories in the overwhelming flood of God's Grace.

Throughout this crippling journey of recovery, Chris became a new man. He found his purpose and voice—not as a victim, but as a survivor and overcomer. The man I know puts people before programs, forgiveness before frustration, healing before hate, and joy before mourning. Chris will be the first to recognize that he is a miracle.

– Dr. Edward Clack D.O

I met Chris Maxwell by "pre-ordained accident." He reached out to me as someone suffering from epilepsy while I was working to change, thinking about this dreadful disease. I didn't know his name on my phone message list, so it languished there for several weeks. When we finally communicated, my life changed. And so did thousands of others. I had a platform with not much to put on it. Chris had a message. Don't give up. Don't give in. Don't doubt yourself. You can make a difference.

I watched him deliver this message in many states in the United States, in Tokyo, Japan, and in South Korea. I watched people of different cultures, experiences, and stages of life all nod in agreement when Chris talked about change and hope and progress. I watched believers and non-believers see a Christlike spirit of love, kindness, and grace encourage them. I witnessed Chris change the lives of hundreds of people across the years . . . just because he had the courage to encourage.

Chris' only tool in this journey was words—words that put just a little piece of himself into their hearts. The piece of himself that said, "It's okay . . . it's all going to be okay." His writing is an extension of Chris, and it will put a little piece of him into your heart as well. Just as I have learned to drink in every minute I get to share with Chris, I encourage you to drink in his words. Just like me, your life will be changed.

– Tom Roberts, Managing Director, UCB

Coming from a near-death, life-threatening medical condition, Chris Maxwell knows firsthand what it is like to feel "underwater," fighting for life. His story is a modern medical wonder and is bringing dignity and hope to people around the world. His voice is being heard at medical conventions, university campuses, and in places of worship. I heartily endorse him and encourage you to have him speak to your organization.

– Dr. A.D. Beacham, Jr., General Superintendent
International Pentecostal Holiness Church

I met Chris Maxwell on the campus of Emmanuel College almost eleven years ago. In our very first conversation, we both knew we had found a friend and even joked about how awesome it would be if we were ever given the opportunity to work together. Be careful what you ask for! We just completed our tenth year working together on the same campus. I never knew the "old" Chris Maxwell, but I read his books, studied his life, and have gotten to know the current Chris extremely well. For many years, we have met weekly to talk, listen, laugh, cry, think out loud, dream, and learn together. We text each other at all hours of the day and night. He can complete my thoughts and finish my sentences. I know his routines, habits, daily rituals, what foods he likes, where he likes to eat, and, often, what he is thinking or feeling. We look out for each other and lean on each other for strength. He is a gift to my life, and I sincerely hope I am a blessing to him as well.

My Chris Maxwell uses words and images to shed light and create life. He thinks, he prays, he writes, and he speaks. His words are well-chosen because they are precious to him. He invests them into our lives strategically in hopes of bringing hope, commonality, mutuality, and trust for a brighter day and better tomorrow. But don't just read the words. Feel the pulse of life, sense the joy in the journey, and embrace the hand of a friend who understands pain, disappointment, temporary setbacks, challenges, hard work, and the routine of daily repetition. Walk with him as he does the sacrificial work of reliving the nightmares of the past as a means of birthing new life and vision for a brighter future for your life. Savor every second and live every moment as if it were all you have. Dive in. Take the plunge. Go deep. Emerge as a better version of you. It can be done. You can learn to live again.

– C. Tracy Reynolds, VP for Student Development
Dean, School of Christian Ministries, Emmanuel College

I remember the day in March 1996 when we received a phone call that our friend and pastor Chris Maxwell was in the hospital, and they weren't sure exactly what was wrong. We came to learn that he was diagnosed with encephalitis which is swelling in the brain. This educated, articulate, and compassionate man had to relearn how to hold a spoon, use the bathroom, and his family's names. All of a sudden, Chris was not the man we knew before. Little did we know the intricate plan God had before him or the people he would meet and touch along the way.

As Chris struggled to learn things all over again, he faced frustrations but also experienced miracles! His healing and accomplishments far exceeded what anyone thought possible! People he might not have ever met if it weren't for his illness were touched by his authenticity and his raw love for God.

The struggles brought Chris further in his faith in a new and fresh way that he may not have reached had he not gone through those physical and mental difficulties.

Today, Chris is educating and inspiring others who have epilepsy. A beautiful picture of how God turns what appears to be a tragedy into blessing, growth, and inspiration for others!

– Marsha Bozeman, Family Nurse Practitioner

I had the pleasure of meeting Chris several years ago when he and I were scheduled to speak at the same program. He is an outstanding speaker! His was a hard act to follow. His talk was extremely well-delivered, inspirational with just the right touch of humor. You find yourself wanting more when the talk ends.

I am equally impressed with Chris' writing ability. It is the kind of writing that makes you think, "I wish I could write like that." He wrote an essay on New Year's Day that I have forwarded to folks all over the country and a few out of the country.

I have seen how Chris relates to people in the audience, the folks who come up to talk to him afterward, and how he seems to instinctively know what they are asking that is not spoken. He is a hero and one the world badly needs. How lucky are those college students who have access to him. What a role model to have at this time in the world.

– Patricia A. Gibson, MSSW ACSW, Associate Professor
Wake Forest University Health Sciences

It was an early morning breakfast appointment. I arrived on time, and my friend who I was going to meet was always early. To my surprise, I beat him to the restaurant. That never happened, but that day it did. I waited on his arrival. My friend and pastor was Chris Maxwell; he never showed. I called and found out later that he was in the hospital with encephalitis. This mysterious disease almost took the life of my friend, but God was gracious. Today, my friend's mind and memory have limitations that did not exist before that day, but his heart has been enlarged, and his sensitivity toward God and others is without measure.

– Tim Kuck, Executive Vice President and C.O.O., Regal Boats

When Chris suffered a debilitating attack of viral encephalitis, he had been my friend, youth pastor, and then pastor for over ten years. I'd met him shortly after moving to the Orlando area when I attended a youth service he was leading. I liked him. Chris was an intellectual and a poet (and still is), and most of all, people were drawn to him and then, through him, to Christ. He was a young, charismatic pastor who used mnemonic devices to memorize the names of every parishioner, spouse, and their children in every congregation with which he associated, and his number one message—a message that he reinforced with his own deacon board and church later on—was the message of God's unconditional love and acceptance. Because of his commitment to that message, I witnessed many broken people over the years receive healing under his ministry, and I saw unconditional commitment extended to so many of us despite our failures and sin. It was unsurprising, then, that when his illness took away his ability to speak coherently that his congregation unconditionally rallied behind him. There wasn't any talk about replacing our pastor even though the prognosis was bleak. And six weeks later, miraculously, he was back in the pulpit. He struggled, but his message was clear. And years later—many years later—he is still writing, speaking, and preaching. I have no doubt that he carries the burden of his illness every day, as does his wife Debbie and his children, but he is now, more than ever, like the high priest of Hebrews who is not unfamiliar with our sufferings. When he writes about faith, suffering, and perseverance, it is because of his own intimate struggle with all three. What you are reading in his words aren't platitudes, but blood and bone and flesh and suffering and the ways that God's love comes to us through all of these.

– Dr. James Rovira, Chair and Associate Professor of English
Mississippi College

Chris Maxwell is a dynamic leader with a message of inspiration. He motivates the masses to live beyond the diagnosis of encephalitis and epilepsy to find their true purpose and calling in life, not by asking "why," but by encouraging others to find their stories of strength. His unique speaking and storytelling is in a league of its own, comprised with compassion and thoughtfulness. Chris invites you into his journey with a tranquil voice and captures your attention with optimistic words that speak to the core of your being. For my personal experience of living with epilepsy, his speaking, writing and stories are the epitome of hope.

– LaKeisha Parnell, Confidence Coach, International Speaker, Author,
Founder of LPForward, LLC

UNDER WATER

When ...

- ENCEPHALITIS,
- BRAIN INJURY and
- EPILEPSY

... Change Everything

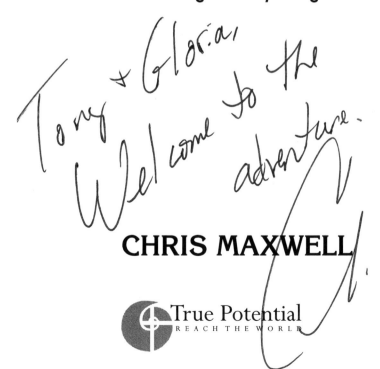

Tony + Gloria,
Welcome to the adventure.

CHRIS MAXWELL

True Potential
REACH THE WORLD

Medical Disclaimer
Underwater contains information related to health care. However, it is not intended to replace medical advice. The author and publisher disclaim liability for any medically related comments that may occur in any stories and ideas from *Underwater* or any references it includes.

Privacy Disclaimer
Most of the names and stories included are accurate. A few names have been changed or are not included, and a few stories have been slightly altered to protect the privacy of those providing their stories.

UNDERWATER
When Encephalitis, Brain Injury and Epilepsy Change Everything

ISBN 978-1-943852-52-9 (Paperback)
ISBN 978-1-943852-53-6 (ebook)

Library of Congress Control Number: 2017934049

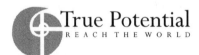

True Potential, Inc
PO Box 904, Travelers Rest, SC 29690
www.truepotentialmedia.com

Printed in the United States of America.

Appreciation and Dedication

As for me, I need to tell a story.[1] —Kathleen Norris

Thank you to my family and friends, my doctors and caregivers, my counselors and accountability partners, my readers and students, my editors and publisher. Life in the plural helps all people—especially those of us who frequently feel singular and lost at sea. This book hopes to honor and encourage all those who have some type of brain damage and often feel that way—*Underwater*. Though memory is difficult for many of us, let's remember we are not alone. Let's remember we are loved. And let's encourage one another to find joy underwater as we endure the adventure.

---

1   Kathleen Norris, *Acedia & me: A Marriage, Monks, and a Writer's Life* (New York: Riverhead Books, 2010) 47.

Contents

Foreword

By Dr. Hal Pineless

I met Chris Maxwell on a Friday afternoon. I was the neurologist at the hospital, and I was finishing hospital rounds when Dr. Adler, the hospital infectious disease specialist, asked me to see Chris. Chris was confused and had a high fever. He spoke nonsensically; had impaired comprehension, and naming. His wife and family couldn't believe the sudden change in Chris' personality.

Chris was a successful Orlando pastor beloved by those whose lives he touched. Chris could remember the name of everyone he met prior to his illness. That changed after Chris was diagnosed with herpes simplex encephalitis. His MRI of the brain looked like Swiss cheese, and I knew it was permanently scarred. Chris was rapidly treated with medications as, luckily, herpes encephalitis was treatable with medicine. Chris developed seizures as a result of his encephalitis, which isn't uncommon. His seizures eventually became controlled with medication.

After hospital discharge, Chris needed extensive rehabilitation. One of Chris' biggest problems was learning to speak, name, and comprehend. The encephalitis destroyed his left temporal lobe, which is important in such functions as memory, naming, expressing emotions, hearing, and auditory processing. Seizures commonly develop in the temporal lobe as well.

Thankfully, Chris was innately stubborn, and this served him well during his rehabilitation. He gradually regained the ability to speak and comprehend. His language skills improved exponentially—nothing short of a miracle.

Now Chris is a prolific author, pastor, radio commentator, and lecturer. He has truly taken a lemon and made it into lemonade. Chris has become a passionate epilepsy advocate, and speaks internationally about his experiences overcoming his illness and epilepsy.

If any neurologist looks at Chris' MRI of the brain and then sees Chris, they can't believe they are looking at the same person. Chris could easily have gone into a deep depression over his illness. His tenacity to stubbornly refuse to lose is what made him into the winner in life that he is today.

I hope that when you read *Underwater: When Encephalitis, Brain Injury and Epilepsy Change Everything*, you will realize that, like Chris, you too have the ability to dominate over your obstacles. Don't let epilepsy or your illness define you. You can succeed in life if you believe in what you are doing and are willing to fight for it. I hope that you will like this book and that it will help you in your journey through life.

Hal S. Pineless, D.O., FACN

President, NeuroCare Institute of Central Florida, Winter Park, FL

Clinical Assistant Professor of Medicine (Neurology)

Florida State University College of Medicine

Medical Director, NeuLife Rehabilitation, Mt. Dora, FL

Introduction: The Song

I had passed from the subject to the direct object of every sentence in my life.[1] —Paul Kalanithi

I have been feeling very clearheaded lately and what I want to write about today is the sea. It contains so many colors. Silver at dawn, green at noon, dark blue in the evening. Sometimes it looks almost red. Or it will turn the color of old coins. Right now, the shadows of clouds are dragging across it, and patches of sunlight are touching down everywhere. White strings of gulls drag over it like beads.

It is my favorite thing, I think, that I have ever seen. Sometimes I catch myself staring at it and forget my duties. It seems big enough to contain everything anyone could ever feel.[2] —Anthony Doerr

I don't know much about life underwater.

But I remember experiences as I glance back in time.

Learning to swim as a kid while Mama watched, smiling. Those fun moments of riding the waves in brief visits to the beach as a child, then as my wife, Debbie, and I were raising our sons. Catching a bonnethead shark by hand—twice—on a vacation with the family. Riding with a dolphin at a theme park. Going on a cruise, visiting the islands of Bequie, Dominica, St. Martens, St. Lucia, and other spots as we noticed beauty at sea and on shore. Snorkeling with Debbie on our trip to Cancun.

The underwater endeavors lure me. The researchers impress me. Their knowledge and experience invite me to investigate. I've dreamed about lengthy periods of time underwater—staring at the gorgeous colors, swimming among the dazzling creatures, slowly adjusting to a new reality.

---

1 Paul Kalanithi, *When Breath Becomes Air* (New York: Random House, 2016) 141.

2 Anthony Doerr, *All the Light We Cannot See: A Novel* (New York: Scribner, 2014) 405.

I've also feared the unknown and the unsafe. I've wondered if I entered the water, would I ever be able to find the boat and come ashore.

But figuratively—and in the context of this book—I actually know much about living underwater. As I wrote in *Changing My Mind*,[3] I know much about remembering less. I know much about being tossed deep below the surface—no advance warning, no prep work, no guidebook, no six weeks of training.

I fell, or rather, was thrown into the ocean. Wearing dress clothes, carrying the luggage of a normal life in our preplanned world, smiling at faces of friends staring back, assuming all was under my own control, I slipped from the safety of a normal life and landed deep in the water.

Would I survive this calamity?

What would life be like before returning to land?

If I did emerge, how different would I then be?

That story and those questions are not about a real ocean. My sea encounter was about my life and my brain and about the lives of those around me changing suddenly through an illness I barely survived.

The underwater image comes from a song Taylor Maxwell, our oldest of three sons, wrote about how he felt as a young man watching his father change.

The word *Underwater* became the title of his song. And since the mood fits where we travel in this book, he gave us permission to use that same title.

How Taylor felt writing the song is a good place for us to begin this journey.

Why did he write the song "Underwater"? "I just wanted to process the emotions of growing up with a dad that had some brain disabilities."

What about your father's illness caused you to feel that way? "It all felt pretty unfair to me. Other than the fact it didn't take his life, I just couldn't understand why so much could be taken from such a good guy. Really, from all of us. The way we all had to do life after he became ill felt so unnatural to me."

When Taylor wrote, "I've been living underwater, on my own and all the time," he "felt in no man's land. The point I was at—growing up as a young man, making my way through high school. It felt lonely."

The song is sad but ends well. How can life stories like ours and those of many others with brain damage end well?

---

3 *Changing My Mind* is Chris' first book that chronicled his recovery from encephalitis.

Taylor says,

> It takes adjusting. I think, especially nowadays, there's this unrealistic drive to reach back in time to the "good ole days," when really the best days can be up ahead. Living in the past is what kills the present. Embracing the present is what shapes the future in new and exciting ways. Life will never be like it was—for anyone. But the amazing thing about life is that we can always be diligent to work towards a more hopeful tomorrow when we breathe deeply in each moment.

Because he is my son, he knows me well. How would he describe ways his dad still feels underwater, two decades after the illness first hit?

> I don't really know, other than how unnatural it is for someone to experience what he did. It's unnatural to be underwater. But once you learn there is a lot to explore there—you can open up new and exciting possibilities. I think he's in that phase. By embracing the incredible challenge, and yet, still moving forward in hopeful exploration.

What can other people do to come up from living underwater?

> There's a work being done in us all underwater. So really, the way I felt writing the song or going through challenging points in life is that you only resurface when the deep underwater work is done.

How can this new book help patients and their caregivers realize they feel underwater while also encouraging them to come up for air and swim onto land?

> It's okay to have an honest assessment of what you're dealing with. Sometimes it takes us identifying others who are in the same situation as we are and being honest with each other. There is a coming ashore moment when you honestly embrace the new you.

What can this book do to help others take those steps to recovery?

> Stay in the moment. Let the present struggle do its good work in you.

Yes, it felt strange interviewing my own son about my life, about his life, about our lives, about the life underwater of so many people. But even through the terror underwater, we've remembered to love. We've chosen to endure. And we have helped each other in the process.

Another person remembers the old me and the new me, the pre-illness Chris and the post-illness Chris. I served as Mary DeMent's pastor as my life almost ended—as the life I had known did end. Her comments come from her lenses as a counselor and a friend:

> To me, Chris is more than fine considering what he has been through. I tell my friends that they would not notice any difference. And it's true. Those who don't have regular contact with Chris would probably not detect any changes in his behavior, his sermon delivery, etc.

> Sometimes, though, I notice subtle changes. For instance, Sunday. He struggled reading a certain word during his sermon. The word was posted on an overhead PowerPoint presentation. Something he never used. He held sermon notes. Something he never did. He wiped his mouth repeatedly. Like a nervous habit. Something he never had.

> He struggles to remember names, not faces. Addresses, not places. Most middle-aged people can relate. But not Chris. He never, ever, struggled in that way. He would deliver his entire sermon, including lengthy portions of Scripture, note-free.

> I often wonder the toll his memory loss has had on him. When someone we know dies, we grieve. We cry, doubt, bargain, and later accept. Surely, he must grieve the loss of the skills he once possessed.

> I wonder what stage of grief he is going through, or does he go in and out? It must be difficult. Sometimes he talks about it; most times, from my vantage point, he keeps the pain to himself.

In *Underwater*, some of the grief will come out. Some of the pain will be released.

Please join me on the voyage into my own Neverland, my own Narnia, my own life underwater. Find yourself and your own story within my story and the stories of others. Be honest about yourself. Know yourself well.

And listen.

Listen to deep hurts and large hopes. Listen to reluctance, but dive in anyway. Listen to voices condemning you, and silence them. Listen to voices encouraging you, and receive them.

And listen for a song. A new version of an old song. A song about you—your past and your future, your pain and your pleasure, your wounds and your healing, your limps and your blessings. Listen to it. Learn it. Sing it.

While staring at the gorgeous colors, swimming among the dazzling creatures, and slowly adjusting to a new reality, embrace the wonder underwater.

1

Surprises

Encephalitis is a thief. . . . [It] has quietly been at work for hundreds of years, robbing families of their loved ones, and even in those families where the person survives, it robs them of the person they once knew. Encephalitis steals survivors' capacity to remember as well as their personalities and the types of abilities we generally take for granted: memory, concentration, attention, thinking, judgment, inhibition. For many, there are additional outcomes such as epilepsy and levels of fatigue so great that returning to work or education will remain elusive. This is, of course, where the person survives; many don't.[4] —Ava Easton

The human brain is the most complex of organs—an intricate network of some 200 billion nerve cells and a trillion supporting cells. The brain controls all bodily activity, from heart rate and movement to emotion and learning.[5] —Diane Roberts Stoler, EdD

Goodbyes can be painful.

We shook hands. We hugged. We laughed. We promised to continue dialogue.

I was waving goodbye to family. Not a biological family. Friends I've known for a decade. Fellow partners in this adventure this book calls "underwater."

---

4   Ava Easton, *Life After Encephalitis: A Narrative Approach* (New York: Routledge, 2016) 4.
5   Diane Roberts Stoler and Barbara Albers Hill, *Coping With Mild Traumatic Brain Injury* (New York: Avery, 1998, 7.

Together we've told stories and enjoyed meals and shed tears. Our adventures of life with epilepsy have felt like swimming through oceans of deep water, fierce currents, and unknown surroundings. I'll tell a few of their stories in this book.

I was excited about my plans for the evening, but on that afternoon, I was ready for a nap. Though exhausted from a few days of learning more about epilepsy and spending time with that family, the goodbyes felt like those who fully understood me were leaving. Part of the need for a nap was my brain's yearning to recover from its ongoing endeavor of overwork. Part of the need was a feeling of grief.

Did You Know?

Epilepsy affects over 3 million Americans of all ages—more than multiple sclerosis, cerebral palsy, muscular dystrophy, and Parkinson's disease combined.

source: cureepilepsy.org/aboutepilepsy/facts.asp

Healthy grief. A realization that grieving well is good. When saying goodbye, when departing from those who fully understand you, when swimming from the underwater life you've become familiar with to the life ashore that others find fun, a type of grief is good.

I skipped the hotel elevator and chose the steps. I smiled with appreciation. I shed a few brief tears not knowing when I would see those friends again and remembering those whose health problems have ended their lives.

I took a nap.

When I woke up, I was thinking about this book and those friends. I was waiting for my wife, Debbie, to arrive. I was reaching for the computer to write and thought of these words: *We never said goodbye.*

At first, I tried to think which friend with epilepsy I missed telling goodbye. As I often do, I struggled to remember.

Then I realized the thought wasn't about that weekend or those friends. It was about my adventure underwater. It was about the abrupt invasion of an illness into my life, into the life of my family and friends. It was about what happened in March 1996. It was about the man that I was and the man that I am—two very different guys in so many ways.

We never said goodbye to that me.

I wanted to talk to him—the former Chris.

I would be surprising Debbie later that day as I took her to a nice restaurant by the water in Atlanta, and I thought, *Wouldn't it be nice for her to see again that former me, that pre-illness me, that me she met, that me she married, that me she lost? She never said goodbye to him.*

Would she enjoy dinner better with that me instead of this me?

But she can't. She will arrive and have dinner with me, a man with epilepsy.

Do you know about that word? Do you know about how many of us with epilepsy feel underwater?

Epilepsy is derived from a Greek word, meaning "to possess, seize, or hold." That meaning isn't Greek to the three million Americans experiencing epilepsy. Most feel possessed, seized, or held back. As I battle with epilepsy, I play with the word instead of letting it play with me. Can't those of us with epilepsy choose to possess, seize, and hold our days? Sure we can—because there's hope. For me, hope means that there are effective treatments and ways you can control your epilepsy and live your life.

But too many people who face epilepsy are trying to endure their experience without hope. They feel alone and isolated. They don't understand their medical options and they struggle to seek the best care that is available. While governments and cultures argue various opinions about health care, individuals and families are concerned about seizures, about side-effects of medications, about driving a car, about getting enough sleep, about life.

And the numbers of people living with epilepsy and brain damage continue rising.

Think. Fifteen seconds. They race as you read these words. During that quick moment, one person in America sustained a traumatic brain injury.

Total numbers? Over 1.5 million Americans sustain a traumatic brain injury each year. And 80,000 of us experience onset of long-term disability following those injuries. These statistics reveal a large, confused, sad audience.

For that audience, we offer *Underwater*. We offer narratives and ideas. We use authenticity to pursue community. We might have more questions than advice, but we want readers to say goodbye to the silence about epilepsy. We want readers to say hello to an honest discussion about the adventure underwater—the condition and what all it brings. And we want readers to find—amid the stories of pain and uncertainty and seizures and medications and side-effects and naps and needing help from friends—hope. A positive perspective no matter what else we face. A sense that good days await. A certainty that we aren't alone.

As you read, notice your own life. Through my story and the stories of others, think about your story. Begin believing like never before that the next chapter of your story will bring a few smiles. Believe those smiles can begin now.

- Epilepsy affects over 3 million Americans of all ages—more than multiple sclerosis, cerebral palsy, muscular dystrophy, and Parkinson's disease combined.
- In America, epilepsy is as common as breast cancer and takes as many lives.
- Almost five hundred new cases of epilepsy are diagnosed every day in the United States.
- Epilepsy affects 50 million people worldwide.
- One in one hundred people will develop epilepsy.
- One in ten people will suffer a seizure in their lifetime.
- This year, another 200,000 people in the U.S. will be diagnosed with epilepsy.
- Each year, over 125,000 to 150,000 are newly diagnosed with epilepsy.
- Thirty percent of those diagnosed are children.
- Epilepsy can develop at any age and can be a result of genetics, stroke, head injury, and many other factors.
- For many soldiers, suffering traumatic brain injury on the battlefield, epilepsy will be a long-term consequence.
- In two-thirds of patients diagnosed with epilepsy, the cause is unknown.
- In over 30 percent of patients, seizures cannot be controlled with treatment.
- Uncontrolled seizures may lead to brain damage and death.
- Up to 50,000 Americans die each year from seizures and related causes.
- The mortality rate among people with epilepsy is two to three times higher than the general population.

- Risk of sudden death among those with epilepsy is twenty-four times greater.

- Epilepsy results in an estimated annual cost of $15.5 billion in medical costs and lost or reduced earnings and production.

- Historically, epilepsy research has been under-funded. Each year NIH spends $30 billion on medical research, but just one half of one percent is spent on epilepsy.

- The Federal government spends much less on epilepsy research compared to other diseases, many of which affect fewer people.

Don't be possessed, seized, or held back.

Seize the moment.

This moment.

That is what many of us are trying to do. As I am trying, I hear many questions still running through this damaged mind.

What is it like saying goodbye to a person who is still alive? What is it like never being able to say goodbye to that person, never being able to grasp or grieve their loss? You knew him or her—or yourself—well. Now you are learning about and accepting the new self or spouse or parent or child or friend or coworker. Now you are trying to learn them. Now you are trying to accept them. You are trying to know them—why they do what they do, how they feel, what you should do, how you feel. You are trying to learn and accept and know you.

> ### What's Helped Me
> - Rest well and often.
> - Drink water.
> - Exercise. If walking is all you can do, walk gladly.
>
> *Chris Maxwell*

Should you help them complete the sentence or remember the name? Should you, as the patient, let those around you locate that word hiding in an unnoticed location in the damaged brain?

Or maybe this is the only you—epilepsy has always been a part of your life.

This isn't a collection of easy answers. It offers ideas but is mainly a confession of the adventure many of us endure. Each day. Each moment. Each word we work to remember.

This is my effort to adjust to the new me.

This is our effort to adjust to the new us.

So welcome to the journey of hidden mysteries and moments of desperation. Welcome to an adventure of pursuing shore while seeking rest amid the unknown. Welcome to swimming among waves in the deep. Welcome to firm rocks, unexpected shallow water, and a sight of unfamiliarity staring back. Welcome to the cold—of numb hands and feet and faces. Welcome to inner questions of endurance or surrender. Welcome to turbulence of fatigue, exhaustion. Welcome to the existence of feeling warn out, swimming with an ongoing desire to be back in bed. Welcome to the overwork of the brain's functioning region that seeks to pick up the slack from the damaged portion's inability to do its tasks. Welcome to confessions of how the brain battles events like its own versions of tsunamis, ridges, valleys, slopes, trenches, shelves, seamounts, cliffs, caves, arches, stacks, terraces, currents, and lagoons. Welcome to coming ashore to an unknown beach. Welcome to the world of disease and disability, the world of encephalitis and epilepsy, the world of scar tissue, the world of seizures and medication, the world of an electrical system under construction until forever.

Welcome to life *Underwater*.

Did You Know?

In America, epilepsy is as common as breast cancer and takes as many lives.

source: cureepilepsy.org/aboutepilepsy/facts.asp

2

Storms

This book is a meditation forwards and backwards over the losses and gains that accompany long-term illness. Some of its pieces follow one another like chapters in a novel, others connect more associatively, like poems in a collection. It is finally an account of change and, I think, growth.[6] —Floyd Skloot

Temporal lobe epilepsy, or TLE, consists of seizures in a part of the brain controlling feelings and memories. During the TLE seizure, a person is overtaken by powerful emotions, usually anger or fear, by hallucinatory voices or visions, or by a vivid flashback. The seizure lasts moments or minutes, rarely more than an hour, and it is accompanied by no apparent physical change, except sometimes a dull stare or a trembling of the arm or mouth. During the seizure, the person may move about as if sleepwalking and may perform automatic acts, sometimes violent, which she is later unable to recall. Unlike the far better known seizures . . . TLE seizures are not easily recognized.[7] —Eve LaPlante

Tell me your name. I'll try to remember it.

But I won't.

I'll forget it. Quickly.

---

6   Floyd Skloot, *The Night-Side: The Chronic Fatigue Syndrome and the Illness Experience* (Ashland, OR: Story Line Press, 1996) xiv.

7   Eve LaPlante, *Seized: Temporal Lobe Epilepsy as a Medical, Historical, and Artistic Phenomenon* (New York: HarperCollins, 2000) 1–2.

I know all the memory tricks. I've tried them. They worked for me before March 1996. Since then, the tricks do not work. Much of my brain doesn't work.

I forget. I strategically plan a variety of techniques to remember. I remember for a moment, a brief moment. Soon I forget again. The rhyme, the image, the melody, the association: scar tissue in my left temporal lobe doesn't follow the rules of those games.

I hear leaders talk about how forgetting someone's name reveals poor leadership. I hope they do not learn the way I learned about forgetting, about brain damage, about epilepsy.

But what I do remember is like a storm that permanently damaged the world of my mind, my emotions, my life. Come for a few moments and visit the storm with me.

Looking back to March 1996, I remember some parts of the story. I'd been going about a normal life adventure and had a headache one day; those weren't typical for me. My wife, Debbie, was alarmed when I slept through a breakfast appointment the next day. Then I started seeing things and saying weird things like, "Your rabbits ran into the house," to my sons, who had no rabbits. I behaved oddly for a few days—until Debbie took me to the hospital.

The headache and visions turned out to be encephalitis, a swelling of the brain caused by an infection. The resulting brain damage and scar tissue would change my personality, affect my memory, and lead to a diagnosis of epilepsy.

That began my voyage underwater.

I spent ten days in the hospital, hallucinating, as the doctors worked to treat me. Once, in the middle of the night, I decided I'd been there long enough and undid the tubes keeping me tied to the hospital bed. I walked out of my room wearing only my shirt. I went down the long hallway and up to the nurse's station. I stood before the calmly panicking nurse saying words—thinking they made sense. She quickly called for my nurse to return me to my room.

My brain wasn't functioning correctly—and I didn't know it.

Have you ever felt scared of what your brain was doing without you knowing it?

As the swelling in my brain went down, it became obvious that some of my memory had been lost. It was like my hard drive had been wiped clean of some of the most basic information. I had to learn to eat, to talk, and to live all over again.

While attempting to eat spaghetti with my fingers, I complained, "This is messy." Debbie handed me a fork and said, "Try using this."

I tried some cold, white stuff from a bowl. I stuttered my excitement to Debbie, saying, "This is good!"

"Yes," she calmly replied, "It's ice cream. You like it."

When Debbie vowed for better or for worse, in sickness and in health, did she ever imagine I'd one day be so clumsy, so crude, or so childish?

But some things didn't change: I still hated onions. Debbie watched me pick them out of the hospital meatloaf and wondered what would be the same and what would change in our lives.

Some of these challenges were humorous, but others were difficult. It seemed that the scholarly Chris was reborn as a friendlier, more caring, more forgetful version. I became a better listener, partly because I had to—there was so much to learn. I could recognize some people but not say their names. I couldn't even remember the names of my three sons when I was in the hospital.

And when my father came to visit me, I didn't call him "Pops." I smiled, though. He turned and walked away, crying.

What's Helped Me

• Do not procrastinate.

• Write to remember, to release emotions, to think, to remind someone you care for them.

Chris Maxwell

My sisters came. My friends came. My staff came. But who was the me they saw there?

After that life-threatening hurdle, it was time to face a season of life underwater: living with epilepsy. As I recovered, I'd have skips in my memory or my mind would wander, and people attributed my forgetfulness to the results of my encephalitis—but I was having partial seizures frequently. It was hard to distinguish between epilepsy and memory loss, but as my mind recovered, the seizures became more noticeable. So, after many tests, another journey began— one that included epilepsy and learning about how other people live with it.

I've come to accept that I must live with epilepsy. But today, I know that I'm not alone. You're not alone either. If we're all here today, we're at least surviving epilepsy—and I think you must have hope, too.

My desire to live a full life with epilepsy is based on a hope that I've seen grow. People with epilepsy have come a long way, especially in how we treat it. I've taken a variety of anti-epileptic drugs since being diagnosed with epilepsy, and I had a variety of side effects.

At one point in my journey, I felt like I'd just "had enough" with too many ineffective drugs, so I sat down with my doctor for a serious talk. My neurologist found what he thought would work best for me, and he was right. I'm so grateful because I found the medication that helped me have seizure control without noticeable side effects.

Did You Know?

Almost five hundred new cases of epilepsy are diagnosed every day in the United States.

source: cureepilepsy.org/ aboutepilepsy/facts.asp

Finding the right medication for all patients with epilepsy is important. Don't take it lightly. As you all know, we're all different. Our bodies react to medications and treatments differently. So what works for me might not work for you or your friend who has epilepsy, and it's a personal decision you should sit down with your doctor to talk about.

When you are talking to your doctor, make sure that you are communicating openly and honestly about these types of things. After all, doctors aren't mind-readers—and a good doctor will be willing to work with you on your treatment goals. Sometimes it's hard to remember things—believe me, I know. If you need help, find someone to go with you to appointments.

The scar tissue that causes my seizures will always be there, but I can control the seizures with medication. Occasionally, I still have auras—perceptual disturbances that signal the onset of a seizure—especially when I travel or have too much in my schedule. If I am traveling, I set an alarm so I can remember my medication. I also make sure to take naps when I need them and try to pace myself.

These days, I keep all the information I need in my iPhone. I write things down; I actually write almost everything down. And whenever someone comes to my office, my staff makes sure to say the person's name to me right before he or she enters.

Despite all the unexpected changes and the pain of this life that often feels underwater, I'm loving where my journey has taken me. These words and sentences will let you visit my story and the stories of others—the underwater encounters we faced and continue to experience.

All I've learned has brought me to this conclusion: We must be open to real experiences, no matter how painful they are. We must process those experiences and, in the end, share them. I tell you my story, not just to make you laugh or cry, but to allow myself to admit that it's been a hard and complicated road for my family and me—my wife, who had a get to know a very different husband, and my sons, who suddenly had to deal with a new father.

But I am not alone. There are over three million of us in the United States alone—more than multiple sclerosis, cerebral palsy, muscular dystrophy, and Parkinson's disease combined. And there are about five hundred new cases of epilepsy diagnosed each and every day.

So I write for them, for you. For the many who battle the consequences of encephalitis and the life with epilepsy. For the many who face underwater encounters from other causes with just as painful effects. For the many who still seek ways to come up from the deep to find air, to find healing, to find hope, to find a friend.

And I write for me. When I'm teaching, I encourage my students to write for the health of it—to get those emotions out—and sometimes, I have them write the stories of their futures. For all of us with epilepsy, I envision a better future with fewer seizures and more understanding, where everyone can be honest about their struggles. Maybe you've heard that "the truth shall set you free." I've been able to explore the truth of who I was, admit the hardships of my experience, and accept the new life I've been given. Now, I want you to explore this adventure with me.

3

Scars

Sometimes the most important questions, those that float in vague suspension for much of our lives, can crystallize in a single moment.[8] —Philip Yancey

Because of the complexity of the brain, epilepsy, to an extent like no other disease, is about individuals: each seizure experience is unique, and each person is touched by it in very different ways. Not only do the different areas of the brain have very different functions, but everyone's brain is wired in a unique manner.[9] —Carl W. Bazil, MD, PhD

Staring at a screen is normal in our image-driven culture. But on that early morning in a dim room, I gazed at an image which proved to not be normal.

White gray segments revealed a problem—just their appearance differed from the darker portions considered correct. The how-it-shouldn't-look depiction was a visual reminder of me and my struggle to remember.

Before my eyes looked at the computer screen, revealing realities of the world within my skull, I lay down for thirty-five minutes—not allowed to move, only breathing and praying and thinking while feeling and hearing forceful percussion. Trapped in that place of investigation and revelation, I rested. I actually felt peaceful in that peculiar cabinet; instead of seeing it as a test to reveal my condition, I had learned to embrace it for a Sabbath.

---

8   Philip Yancey, *Disappointment with God: Three Questions No One Asks Aloud* (Grand Rapids, MI: Zondervan Books, 1988) 35.

9   Carl W. Bazil, *Living Well with Epilepsy and Other Seizure Disorders: An Expert Explains What You Really Need to Know* (New York: HarperCollins, 2004) 12.

I recalled previous MRIs (magnetic resonance imaging). I wondered if the damage to my brain would be the same or worse or better. I remembered when encephalitis initiated all these tests and almost caused my life on earth to end. My thoughts traveled in circles from past to present to future—all while waiting to view the latest news on my brain.

This brain of mine—scars creating crafty artwork through the left temporal lobe—needs to settle on a thought. If it wavers too soon it might never return. Repetition and concentration and simple instructions help its ability to grasp, to maintain, to understand, to retain, to explain. On that day, and in that passageway of exploration, my thoughts dwelled only on themselves for a while as the MRI's back-and-forth rhythms continued exposing their effort to know me well.

So I settled on thoughts about thinking. About my brain, though severely damaged, still an astonishing work of design. About the brain's parts, all team players hoping to win. About the brain's weaknesses when damaged, something I know well. About the methods of recollection, seeking to hold on to a noun or a number or an encounter or a person before escaping into my land of forgetfulness. While a magnetic field and radio waves labored for useful diagnostic information, I just thought. While not able to move at all, I just thought about thinking—of these mysteries we are, of these brains at work, of these methods of remembering.

So much, really, is cooperation. Human bodies toil as a team of many parts. Nineteen muscles partner just to move a hand and wrist.

> **What's Helped Me**
> • Look in the mirror, and believe the person looking back is important.
> • Forgive those who have hurt you. Refuse to let pains from the past control your present and future decisions.
> *Chris Maxwell*

According to "50 Amazing Human Brain Facts (Based on the Latest Science)"[10] by Deane Alban, the brain is capable of some amazing things. Here are just a few:

- The typical brain is about 2 percent of a body's weight but uses 20 percent of its total energy and oxygen intake.

- Your brain is 73 percent water. It takes only 2 percent dehydration to affect your attention, memory and other cognitive skills.

- Each neuron connects with, on average, 40,000 synapses.

- A piece of brain tissue the size of a grain of sand contains 100,000 neurons and 1 billion synapses all communicating with each other.

- Brain information moves between 1 mph and an impressive 268 mph, faster than Formula 1 race cars which top out at 240 mph.

My interaction with my other family— people who experienced encephalitis; patients who live with epilepsy—has helped me understand more than facts about the brain. We've had to learn—not wanted to learn, but learned in desperation, in survival— how we learn, why we forget, what triggers seizures, and how those mesmerizing brain facts leave out portions of our lives. We've learned words and phrases, and though we forget them or struggle to spell them, we relate to their importance: synapses, electrical impulses, transmitter molecules, synchronicity, circuit, embedded, forming of memory, trace, frequency embedded, rebuilding, face recognition, neurons, network, retract, regenerating, frail, stress, post-synaptic neuron, molecules, caregivers, rest, meditation, fragile, errorless learning.

Did You Know?

Epilepsy affects

50 million people

worldwide.

source: cureepilepsy.org/ aboutepilepsy/facts.asp

Those words come and go, appear and disappear, approach and depart when I seek to explain my brain and its scar tissue to others. When I hope to make sense of my failure to make sense, I often fail. But I remember some of what I'm forgetting. I remember the brain's fascinating facts and its goal

---

10   Deane Alban, "50 Amazing Human Brain Facts (Based on the Latest Science)," https://bebrainfit.com/human-brain-facts/ accessed December 17, 2016.

to partner with all the portions of itself. I remember how, when some parts are unable to function correctly, other portions work hard, often overwork, to function correctly.

I then remember words Paul Kalanithi wrote in his book *When Breath Becomes Air*: "I began to realize that coming in such close contact with my own mortality had changed both nothing and everything."[11]

I can relate.

If a scholar becomes a poet, if a teacher becomes a storyteller, if a doctor becomes an artist, if an athlete becomes a friend, if the one bringing healing becomes the one in need, what has really changed? Just the brain? Or everything?

As the brain in my head changed, I changed. The Chris who remembered became the Chris who forgets. The temporal lobe scar tissue could no longer correctly house and distribute the material I depended on for life and career: words. Names refused to appear in ways accessible. Sentences stopped midstream. Moods mixed and mingled and merged. Vision blurred. Silence took up residency in dialogue.

My new nouns of life became words like seizure, nap, mood, memory, medication. My new moods became extremes from peace to madness, before finding balance with the help of rest and rules and medical advice and prayer and medication. My family remembers how I changed—quickly, painfully, permanently.

My neurologist remembers the cause as he explains the effect. I still hear Dr. Hal Pineless saying, "You now have epilepsy." He's the same one who used humor to help me smile, saying, "Remember what Clint Eastwood says in the Dirty Harry movies: 'A man's got to know his limitations.'"

Isn't that word *limitations* a curse? How can I view it as a blessing? I asked Dr. Pineless for more information about my battle, my war, my struggle.

He said, "You would vary between having a hard time remembering what you wanted to say, getting frustrated when you couldn't say it, and then sometimes just talking gibberish. Over time, that started going away. When I began seeing you in the office, you felt frustration that you couldn't express what you wanted to say."

"One of the things that affected you," Dr. Pineless said, "and still does, is names. The area where you're damaged is the *naming center* of the brain. I

---

11 *When Breath Becomes Air*, 131.

remember hearing that you could remember names easily before. Now you still have to use devices and look at people you work with who can help you know a person's name."

He describes for me what I have learned from experience and for research to know myself better. He says, "The most common types are partial complex or temporal lobe seizures. That's where your injury is: in the left temporal lobe. You might do things like staring off into space. People could be talking, and you wouldn't really be connected with the environment. Or I've had some people tell me they're aware of what's going on, but they can't communicate. Or they may do unusual things like start picking things off the wall that aren't there. That's part of the seizure."

His words help me understand my lack of understanding.

Another key word for me—and for all of us members of the brain-damaged tribe—is *hope*. Individuals and groups need that word. My brain remembers it; I can spell it and talk about it. In some odd ways, my mental adventure underwater has helped me live with hope.

Neurological adventures, anti-epileptic medications and their side effects, inner wars, words hiding in the let-me-house-your-nouns-until-you-need-them section of the brains, numb hands, numb feet, slow methods of processing how to answer an unexpected but simple question, and an exhausted electrical system in need of a nap when others want to run marathons—those realities could cause sadness. Sometimes they do. But as I stare at the MRI results, I remember. I actually do remember. One word. One four-letter word. Hope.

Hope to continue. Hope in the brain and the Designer of that craftwork. Hope in hope—to live and breathe, to smile and care, to endure and not give up, to say the word *epilepsy* and spell it correctly, to believe, to continue this voyage.

Kathleen Norris wrote about that four-letter word: "But hope has an astonishing resilience and strength. Its very persistence in our hearts indicates that it is not a tonic for wishful thinkers but the ground on which realists stand."[12]

---

12   Kathleen Norris, *Acedia & Me: A Marriage, Monks, and a Writer's Life* (New York: Riverhead Books, 2010) 221.

Instead of dwelling on the scar tissue's disruption of the brain's ideal design, I recall those conversations when staring at my test results. The MRI revealed reality—often hidden, but now on a screen visible for my eyes to see. Clear enough for my brain to understand. Raw enough for even me to remember.

A screen of scars. A revelation of reality. A narrative by image. A case by science.

A brain—created artistically, though damaged now, though unable to function as intended, though wounded. The electrical system fascinates, finds, labors, and, at times, overreacts in an action known as seizures. But, through even that, the art amazes me. Cells are determined to work hard and well and together, even if sometimes they work too hard. Medication and conversations and writing help this scarred brain to see more than the gray. It notices a quest abounding in hope among the storms.

And that hope allows me to sometimes lie down and be still, even when not being tested for the latest revelation of damage. To ride the waves. To rest in the underwater adventure. To hear of hope and breathe. To notice the images all around and appreciate the wonder of now.

What's Helped Me

• Do not assume forgiving means approving of improper behavior. Do not accept harm (physically or verbally) from someone else. Get away from them. But do not let bitterness travel with you.

Chris Maxwell

4

Seizures

All the waves behind them seemed to take on unusual shapes and the sea was a drab or yellowish color like dirty canvas. The air grew cold.[13] —C.S. Lewis

Neurons can be entrained by a variety of nonelectrical stimuli, including light and sound; these effects can be demonstrated using an EEG. Many kinds of sensory stimulation can radically alter the frequency of brain waves. For example, in a hyperexcitable brain, as in some cases of photosensitive epilepsy, strobe lights (flashing at about ten times a second) can cause large numbers of neurons to fire synchronously; a victim may have a seizure, lose consciousness, and start writhing out of control. Music can cause seizures as well.[14]
—Norman Doidge, MD

Imagine life with epilepsy. Consider yourself among us—one of the statistics. Though each person living with epilepsy is different, select a seizure type, choose a cause, pick a particular damage in your brain.

Stare at the server as you sit at your favorite restaurant—with music playing and the smell already tasting delicious—while you can't locate the words in your brain to voice your order. She waits. You search. Friends at the table stare. How do you feel?

---

13 C.S. Lewis, *The Voyage of the Dawn Treader*, The Chronicles of Narnia (New York: Harper Collins, 1952) 71.
14 Norman Doidge, *The Brain's Way of Healing: Remarkable Discoveries and Recoveries From the Frontiers of Neuroplasticity* (New York: Penguin Books, 2016) 346.

Sit in your normal chair for the business meeting with your corporate team. You know the drill. It's your turn. This is your area of expertise; you own it. But this time the words aren't as clear. You slightly stutter, staring at the computer screen. Your hands twitch. Your eyes blink. You begin to sweat. The team waits for your response. How do you feel?

Stand in front of the crowd to perform your favorite solo. You've embraced the scene for a decade. The band plays; you get ready to change the audience's mood with your voice. But the first lines don't flow. You're dizzy. You're not sure if this is real or a dream. The last thing you remember is looking away from the flickering light—its glare was so bright. Soon you're being picked up from the floor and taken to an ambulance. You thought the seizures were gone. Now it seems like the life you love is gone. How do you feel?

Walk around the house. You live alone. Neighbors speak. They'll come by if you call. But no family nearby. No true friends. You wish someone else knew how many seizures you've had the last month. You wish someone was there to remind you what your doctor said in your previous appointment. But you just look out the widow, watching how others appear to be "living life." How do you feel?

> **What's Helped Me**
> • Find the right person to talk to: counselor, life coach, mentor, pastor, friend.
> • Schedule times of relaxation—don't wait to see if they show up.
> • Dream big.
> • Be faithful in everyday tasks, and find pleasure during the routine.
>
> *Chris Maxwell*

Imagine having a seizure during class in middle school. Puberty. Competition for popularity. Body and emotions and beauty and friends. And now this. How does that define your teenage identity?

Imagine preparing a year for a vacation. You've always desired to visit Ireland. Your family heritage seems to have invited you there. You've saved the money and finalized your flights. But the seizures return. More severe than normal. The doctors and your family are concerned. Your trip is cancelled. You'll be enjoying an MRI and an EEG instead of music and food in a place of your dreams.

Dreams? Dream of your driver's license being taken from you. Dream of your body, formerly healthy, feeling exhausted no matter how much sleep you had. Dream of your sweetheart slowly appearing not quite as interested as she was previously—she rarely makes eye contact; those kisses aren't the same; her role appears more like a chore than a romance. Dream of staring at a book and wrestling to understand the meaning of words that you yourself previously wrote. Dream of attention lasting—only that long. Dream of forgetting names and directions and numbers and the most important events of your life story. Dream of causing an accident because of a seizure. Dream of severe side-effects of anti-epileptic medications—weight problems, mood problems, panic problems, numbness, exhaustion, staring. Dream of listening in as all your friends talk, realizing none of them are including you in the conversation. Dream of everyone being invited to the party—everyone but you. Dream of suddenly losing that talent you worked so hard to craft, to develop, to perfect. Dream of hearing your family talk about their difficulties because of your situation—their honesty coming out because they didn't know you could hear them from the bedroom; their aggravation released because they were sure you had already fallen asleep like you normally do at that time each night. Dream of risking your life at war and returning home with traumatic brain injury and epilepsy but hearing no applause, no appreciation, and no support. Dream of forgetting, of fearing, of expecting the worst. Dream of getting the news about a friend with epilepsy dying unexpectedly and always wondering when it might be you.

Did You Know?

One in one hundred people will develop epilepsy.

source: cureepilepsy.org/ aboutepilepsy/facts.asp

Are those pleasant dreams?

Nightmares?

I asked you to imagine because those are some of our encounters. Those are our adventures at sea. Underwater, we aren't sure if we'll remember your name or our most recent conversation or you. We aren't certain how long we'll remain seizure-free—if we're fortunate enough to be one of those. We aren't sure if our anti-epileptic medication will work well—or what the side effects might be. We aren't sure how to pay for next month's medication. We aren't sure when the energy will return, if ever. We aren't sure. That's us, so often. We just aren't sure.

Maybe you relate in a different way. Maybe the bright lights don't bother you, but the painful memories of past relationships just won't leave you alone. Maybe words like exhaustion, fear, confusion, forgetting, hurt, and alone apply to you because of different reasons. Maybe you remember being abused by a parent. Maybe you remember harming yourself and living through it. Maybe you remember taking a business risk after the motivational speaker inspired you, but now you are still suffering financially because of it. Maybe he left you. Maybe she wishes you would leave her. Maybe you failed the test, and your family rejects you for not living up to their expectations. Maybe you missed the shot, your team lost the game, and that is all you're remembered for. Maybe you tried school but aren't fit for it. Maybe the food calls you, lures you, demands you to come. Maybe the food forces its way out. Maybe you spend and spend and spend. Maybe you hate. Maybe you quit every time you are near success because choosing to get out is better than not succeeding. Maybe you can't stay in any place long. Maybe the music about hate is your preferred set because it reminds you of your own self-talk. Maybe you want to get back at someone, anyone, for what those other people did to you.

> **What's Helped Me**
>
> • If you need to (even if it hurts your ego—I said if you "need to," not if you "want to"), let a family member or trusted friend go with you to the doctor. They can help you remember what to tell the doctor and help you remember what the doctor tells you.
>
> *Chris Maxwell*

Maybe one of those sentences resembles your life underwater.

Maybe one of those feels like a life sentence or a death sentence—you feel no way to escape the submerged season of your life.

Have you talked to anyone about it?

A therapist can help. They will listen to your description of sinking deep. They will ask questions. They will assist you in no longer denying your life underwater. They will comfort you amid the current. They will also help you—often slowly, and after drifts and strong waves—come ashore.

When encephalitis shoved me underwater, I was slow in seeking therapy. My speech therapy helped, but eventually I needed more. I needed help to gain a better view toward life, toward the present and the past and the future.

Those with epilepsy know what a seizure means. We know the stories, the stats, the explanations. We also know it personally.

My ocean was covered with new and harsh realities. Many of us now know these words and phrases too well: encephalitis, epilepsy, traumatic brain injury, confusion, hallucinations, seizures, loss of sensation, fatigue, fever, loss of appetite, malaise, irritability, headache, stiff neck, numbness, loss of memory, behavioral/personality changes, physical weakness, intellectual disability, lack of muscle coordination, vision problems, hearing problems, speaking issues, coma, difficulty breathing, death, paralysis, loss of brain function, problems with speech, amnesia, inability to speak or to understand, mental confusion, difficulty concentrating, inability to create new memories, inability to recognize common things, abnormal laughing and crying, aggression, impulsivity, lack of restraint, persistent repetition of words or actions, balance disorder, blackout, dizziness, fainting, anger, anxiety, apathy, loneliness, dilated pupil, raccoon eyes, unequal pupils, nausea or vomiting, sensitivity to light or sensitivity to sound, slurred speech or impaired voice, persistent headache, a temporary moment of clarity, bleeding, blurred vision, bone fracture, bruising, depression, loss of smell, nerve injury, post-traumatic seizure, ringing in the ears, stiff muscles.

Did You Know?

One in ten people will suffer a seizure in their lifetime.

source: cureepilepsy.org/ aboutepilepsy/facts.asp

What is the list of realities of your ocean?

What are you doing to face them and to pursue recovery?

Who is helping rescue you?

Though much of each life struggle is a journey underwater alone, please do not always swim alone. Please, seek rescue. Please, do not suppose you will always stumble on the shore alone.

Notice the lighthouse. Hear the ship. Detect a swimmer coming to your aid.

Make the call.

Dr. Jill Bolte Taylor, Ph.D., writes in *My Stroke of Insight*, "Recovery, however you define it, is not something you do alone, and my recovery was completely influenced by everyone around me." Her list of needs reminds me how I felt underwater:

- I desperately needed people to treat me as though I would recover completely.
- I needed the people around me to believe in the plasticity of my brain and its ability to grow, learn, and recover.
- My brain needed to be protected and isolated from obnoxious sensory stimulation, which it perceived as noise.
- For my recovery, it was critical that we honor the healing power of sleep.
- I needed people to love me—not for the person I had been, but for who I might now become.
- I needed those around me to be encouraging.
- I needed to know that I still had value.
- I needed to have dreams to work toward.
- It was essential that we challenge my brain systems immediately.
- Offer me only multiple-choice questions and never ask me Yes/No questions.
- I had to define my priorities for what I wanted to get back the most and not waste energy on other things.[15]

---

15 Jill Bolte Taylor, *My Stroke of Insight: A Brain Scientist's Personal Journey* (New York: Plume, 2006) 111–114.

5

Searches

The medication switch was almost as brutal as I feared. . . .
I slipped further into a sludge of exhaustion, dizziness, and
nausea . . . as the dose increased. My vision was blurry every
time I adjusted my gaze and my brain felt as if it were floating
in a directionless fog. . . . Although people surrounded me all
day, I felt completely alone.[16] —Kristin Seaborg, MD

Suffering can, if we let it, make us better instead of worse.[17]
—Eugene H. Peterson

Damaged brains swim recklessly, searching for answers, for words, for
solutions.

People like me often swim frantically, searching for ourselves.

Those searches, as I've suggested, can be helped when we aren't doing the
search alone. Finding ears to hear our stories and hearts to care for us are vital
in our healing.

It is not bad to have a psychologist as a friend and neighbor. Well, sometimes
it's bad—he might always be figuring out what I am thinking. But that's okay.
I won't remember, and he is required to keep it confidential.

Blake Rackley, PsyD, Licensed Clinical Psychologist and Associate Professor
of Psychology, is one of many who has helped me process my life underwater.

---

16 Kristin Seaborg, *The Sacred Disease: My Life with Epilepsy* (Seattle:
    Booktrope, 2015) 227.
17 Eugene H. Peterson, *Leap Over a Wall: Earthy Spirituality for Everyday
    Christians* (San Francisco: HarperSanFrancisco, 1998) 198.

Though his thoughts are related to my condition, think of yourself. How does this relate to you, to your story, to your adventure underwater?

Chris' life is affected in many ways. Life isn't easy when a deep need for sameness and no variability are constant. Things that interrupt Chris' routine are often met with frustration and sometimes words that he doesn't mean to say. When his mind becomes sufficiently focused, little things that break into that concentration cause emotional responses that he wouldn't normally have if he didn't have brain damage. Basically, one of his greatest needs is to live without distraction, singularly focused on whatever task he has at hand.

He has learned to adapt in some situations and to accept that certain events or places are nothing but distractions.

Yet, at the end of the day, Chris has to allow his brain to rest by focusing on one task, which is often writing. He has to associate new people and their names with people from his past to remember their names.

What's Helped Me

- Use modern devices to evaluate and maintain your diet, exercise, budget, time management, medications, and schedules.
- Listen to the sound of silence.
- Breathe deeply and slowly.
- Notice the wonder nearby.

Chris Maxwell

Dr. Rackely tells his students about my brain. Showing them my MRI results, he presents the good news I need to remember myself.

I tell my students that they are looking at a miracle, although a broken one. I point to the areas of the brain that have been affected by the encephalitis and tell that he should not be able to speak or, at times, comprehend speech.

As my friend and a psychologist, what does he see as the most difficult parts as I live with ongoing struggles from brain damage?

Life with brain damage and epilepsy for Chris isn't only about his learning to live with the inability to recall names or names of objects. It isn't just about his need for routine and consistency. It is about those around him learning to live with someone different than they might have known before. While Chris is relational at his very core, it affects those relationships closest to him. His deadlines, his need for an environment free from distraction, and his need for sameness affect those closest to him because they have seen him when his guards are down.

Why does Dr. Rackely think so many people with epilepsy or other life struggles feel underwater? What hinders us from coming ashore and finding life around other people?

For many with epilepsy, they feel life is now limited or that they are broken because of their seizures. They feel trapped by their own minds, so they do not reach out to others. Many do not ask for help or seek other relationships because they are embarrassed, ashamed, and/or depressed. They feel they are drowning in a sea of helplessness because they have lost control of the very things that make us feel empowered: our body and mind. They know that people who are unfamiliar with seizures are often scared when they see them have one. They see the looks when they come out of one, they see the stares, and they see potential relationships disappear before their eyes. They hurt so desperately and desire to just live a normal life. Adolescents will wonder about who would want to date them or who would marry them. Adults will wonder who will take care of

> **Did You Know?**
>
> This year, another 200,000 people in the U.S. will be diagnosed with epilepsy.
>
> source: cureepilepsy.org/aboutepilepsy/facts.asp

them if things get worse and wonder if their spouse will leave them. Many feel trapped because they are no longer able to drive or walk. They feel they are drowning in a sea of constant dependency where the waves are their seizures or disability, and they despair that there will not be a life preserver or a rescue team or a family member or a wife or a husband or a child or a friend to help them. Many fear dependency. Many despise the notion that they have to depend on someone else. Many feel guilty that they have to depend on someone else. Many are angry at God for allowing this to happen. Many feel their faith slip away because they have prayed for a miracle.

I will often use Chris as an example in this case. I remind them that while he is a miracle, he is still a broken miracle.

I read Dr. Rackley's words again. I feel sadness as I am reading about shame and embarrassment, about drowning in a sea of helplessness, about losing control, about the stares, about faith slipping away, about the need for a rescue team.

Miracles, though broken.

We feel unsure.

That reminds me of when a friend's daughter had a few feelings that left her a little unsure:

On the morning of her first day at high school, my daughter was a little nervous. As we snaked along the line of cars depositing students at the front doors, she murmured, "I'm scared." I reassured her that she would be just fine. And then, with a slightly panic-stricken look on her face, she asked, "Did I pee this morning?"

We all know a little of those feelings. Scared. Unsure of the new. Not totally prepared for a new adventure. Not knowing if we went to the restroom.

Not quite ready for the storm.

But all of us need to remember this: storms come. In some form, on some day, in some way, storms come. We want life to be a calm and happy cruise, but the waves become fierce. We become nervous.

Years ago, our family tried to prepare for hurricane Charley hitting us, but we still had no control over the story. The trees fell on the house as we sat listening, praying, and scared.

What is your story? The car accident? The emotional turmoil? The cancer? The addiction? The disability?

Is your storm in the ocean learning to live life with epilepsy?

Or is your storm at sea learning to live life as a caregiver?

My wife, Debbie, knows about more storms than the Florida hurricanes and the Georgia tornados. She also knows about how our lives changed quickly the day she rushed me to the ER:

> "In sickness and in health; 'til death do we part." I listened as the young couple spoke these words of commitment to each other. Choked up a little, I held back tears as I watched my husband lead this bride and groom in their wedding vows. I thought, "Do they really understand what they are saying?" I hope and pray that they did and that when a problem or even a tragedy arose in their marriage that they would remember the words spoken in front of witnesses at their wedding.
>
> Our family understands all too clearly what can happen in life to a family when someone becomes seriously ill. Several years ago, my husband contracted encephalitis. We had three young sons, and our family was turned upside down. My husband was very healthy one day, and horribly sick on the next day. After ten days in the hospital, we brought home a very different man from the one who had entered the hospital. Encephalitis had ravaged his brain and caused irreparable damage. Many changes took place in my husband because of this illness, but one was so drastic that I had to start calling him "My Second Husband." His personality changed. There were remnants of the man I married, but in many ways, he was a different person. His understanding was difficult, communication skills slow, sense of humor totally changed, and many more aspects made him a stranger. I felt as if I had

four sons now. I knew very little about this new man I was living with. As the years have gone by, we have learned how to live and love each other. It has not been easy, but we have stayed committed to each other and dedicated ourselves to the vows we made over three decades ago. We are blessed.

Many times I have been reminded of the words of David in the Psalms that say, "Yea, though I walk through the valley of the shadow of death, I will fear no evil; for thou art with me." How true those words are! God had never left us, nor forsaken us. He has been faithful through situation after situation while the boys were growing up, in our marriage, when He called us to move to another job in another state, and through countless other situations.

Lots of people have asked me how I have been able to do this. How could I stay married to a totally changed man; not the one I married? I say that I believe God intended for us to be married. I believed it back in 1981, and if it was true back then, then I am sure that God did not change His mind. My husband's illness did not take Him by surprise. The Lord knew it would happen when we met. We made a commitment, and those should not be easily broken. We watch daily as families dissolve around us for petty, trivial reasons. Only those who stand fast, keep the commitments they have made to the Lord, and put their trust in Him, will reap the reward.

What's Helped Me

• Keep a list of your medical history and present condition, medications you are taking and medications to avoid, times and dosages of those medications you are taking, names and numbers of people to contact (family, doctors, neighbors, friends, etc.) when needed, and other vital information.

Chris Maxwell

Yes, my wife endured the storm to my brain, to my life, to our family, to our relationship, to her. Neither of us always handled it correctly. But we endured the storm and learned through it. And we are still enduring and still learning.

6

Sentences

Disconnecting from change does not recapture the past. It loses the future.[18] —Kathleen Norris

A moment later she found that she was standing in the middle of a wood at night-time with snow under her feet and snowflakes falling through the air.[19] —C. S. Lewis

"Due to brain injury, he has the mental capacity of a three-year-old."

I heard those words from the TV morning news while eating breakfast at a hotel. I was soon traveling to two events in one city to tell my story. That sentence stayed in my mind.

It is strange what I remember and what I forget.

Due to.

Brain injury.

The mental capacity of a three-year-old.

I stood up and walked to the table for another blueberry muffin.

Sitting back down, I ignored the news and looked at my iPad for that day's presentations.

Mental capacity.

Three-year-old.

---

18 Kathleen Norris, *Dakota: A Spiritual Geography* (Boston, MA: Houghton-Mifflin, 1993) 64.
19 C. S. Lewis, *The Lion, The Witch, and The Wardrobe* (New York: Macmillan Publishing Co, Inc., 1950) 5.

We could take the opening four words of that news report and let it begin many of our stories. Due to brain injury, what next?

What sentences should we use to follow that intro?

What sentences describe or define, instruct or advise, laugh at or cry with, pray for or ignore the victims who live life underwater because of brain injury?

And one word from that sentence reveals the people affected: victims.

But as we read in Debbie's comments in chapter five, as I've read in many of her efforts to not let me notice her pain, and as many of you have read in your caregivers' attempts to survive life underwater, those who care for us patients are also victims.

Did You Know?

Each year, over 125,000 to 150,000 are newly diagnosed with epilepsy.

source: cureepilepsy.org/aboutepilepsy/facts.asp

People with epilepsy aren't the only ones in this story. Think of the caregivers. Think of those in the medical and psychological fields. Think of neighbors and employers and teachers.

It's not easy being us. But it's also not always easy being with us.

Maybe we can't totally change that. But as those living with epilepsy and other health issues, we can remember those around us as we move toward our own recovery.

Though some executives display little compassion, and the horror stories anger me, not all businesses are rude to those employees with brain damage. Coworkers and leaders struggle to adjust. They don't always know what to do. Teachers try to adjust, but their schedules and requirements make it tough. Coaches and politicians and news reporters: We all need to engage in conversations. We all need to learn. That's why information and guidance is helpful for all of us.

That's why it is also helpful to hear from those who give and give and give and give their care. Some give until they have very little left.

I wrote earlier some of my son Taylor's comments. Though I am so grateful for our relationship, I also need to recall his pain. Taylor's love of sports and music, his concerts, his willingness to let me listen to the early drafts of his songs: He accepted this me. And I am thankful.

Taylor says the hardest part for him was that my illness came at the beginning of his teenage years. He wanted and needed a father to show him how to navigate those waters. He says, "The illness sort of took that away from me." "Luckily I still had my dad," he said, "But I missed my father in those years."

How did he feel? "I felt bad for my father and also frustrated at the same time. It was pretty confusing since I was young, and then it just became normal."

Aaron, our middle son, felt the underwater pain deeply. He helped me so much during my recovery—helping me learn new technology which assisted in my recall and my communication, playing ball games with me, and adjusting to this new life. But adjusting can be living constantly in the eye of a hurricane. Aaron remembers how I became "totally different" than his pre-illness dad. He felt scared, and he sensed a need to protect his mother and younger brother. The brain damage and mood swings bothered him more than me living with epilepsy. He remembers the days I was released from the hospital, still adjusting to medications and emotions: "It was like a five-year-old throwing temper tantrums, but with the strength of a man who didn't know how strong he was."

Reading his comments, I cry. I feel guilty for something that was out of my control.

I see why so many families fall apart after a person suffers from TBI. I am thankful for encouraging words and deep prayers many people offered for Aaron, his brothers, and his mother.

And I am thankful Aaron did not give up.

On me. On life.

He now encourages people around the world. He now, though I cry and battle guilt whenever I read words about the pain he endured through my sickness, encourages me.

And causes me to remember more than our bad moments underwater. I can remember the good.

For Aaron, spelling words was never simple. Pre-illness Chris could not understand why a person could not hear the word, learn to spell it, and always recall that correct spelling. Post-illness Chris couldn't spell. So though the brain damage caused relational damage, it also helped me to relate and understand others better.

I would call the words out to Aaron, and he struggled to spell them correctly.

Aaron would call the words out to his brain-damaged father, and I would struggle to spell them correctly.

So we would put the books away and go play basketball.

Underwater, for the patients and the caregivers, is dangerous. It brings bites and attacks and deep wounds.

Underwater, for the patients and the caregivers, can also provide an adventure. To pursue common enjoyment, to engage in simple dialogue each person can understand, to smile, to cry, to learn.

Taylor suggests to caregivers, "Just try to be patient. We will never know what they are going through, and they do not know what we are going through. Like any relationship, you have to try your best to take the road of understanding and humility, and whatever works best in your situation. Find boundaries. It has been pretty rough trying to find my way. Luckily, I've had some really great mentors and friends along the way that have helped mark the path for me and gently correct me when I'm lost."

I'll write more about caregivers in chapter 16. For now, I'll repeat myself as those of us with brain damage often do.

Get help.

Find someone to talk to. Not just anyone, but the right person.

For patients and caregivers, the correct listening ears can help identify an underwater experience and offer guidance toward future phases of the journey.

But sometimes, if we are willing, a counseling session might happen unexpectedly.

Beverly J. Oxley, Ph.D., is a friend. She is a licensed psychologist, registered Play Therapist & Supervisor, and owner & director of Wellsprings Psychological Resources. I often write for her and bring students to learn from her story. That is an easy way for me to get therapy while trying to help someone else.

But I didn't expect the therapy that day. We were planning to talk about other ways I could help her and began walking toward her office. I stopped, staring at a "sandtray"—a therapeutic technique that bypasses the language center of our brains and goes to the creative, non-linguistic part of the brain so that our emotions can be accessed without censor.

I wanted her to explain to me the purpose of a sandtray. Instead, she wanted me to participate in the practice. I resisted. She dared. I stared. She laughed.

I didn't laugh. For some reason, the sandtray both bothered me and intrigued me—kind of like talking about my life with epilepsy and writing a book like this.

I decided to engage in the sandtray.

Dr. Oxley remembers what happened:

In the building phase of the sandtray you sprinkled a large array of crystals all over the tray—some were randomly tossed; some were intentionally placed. When you finished scattering crystals, I asked if there was anything else that needed to go in the tray. You found just what you wanted—a pirate ship which you placed in a corner of the tray.

In the processing phase of the sandtray I asked questions such as, "Are there groups of crystals or are they all a part of a random scattering?" You identified them as groups. I asked where you were in the scene. . . you had intentionally placed a "unique" crystal (unlike all the others) in the corner with the pirate ship. You seemed surprised at the question, but then identified the unique crystal as the one that represented yourself. I asked you to tell me what is happening in that corner of the tray. You explained that you often boarded the pirate ship to travel to various "islands"—going from place to place, spending time at various "islands" but always returning to the corner. When asked if anyone were with you, you replied that most the time you were alone, but at times, Debbie was with you, and sometimes your whole family, but mostly you were alone.

As I recall, the purpose of your travels was mainly for helping others and sometimes to visit your family, but

---

What's Helped Me

• Read. If reading is difficult because of brain damage, listen to the audio version of books and talks. Keep the mind thinking.

Chris Maxwell

---

you always returned to the corner of safety. "Do you ever experience loneliness?" You indicated that indeed you did get lonely at times. Even the presence of family and friends didn't allay the loneliness, but you seemed to find contentment in your solace.

What do I see as a therapist? I see that you find meaningful work to do to keep you from feeling lonely and unconnected. It seems that social engagements just for the sake of social activity is not satisfying to you. Perhaps this is the "underwater" feeling of isolation . . . others appear to you to be out of the water—enjoying life on the beach, playing, eating, drinking, socializing, but you feel as if you are in a large ocean filled with islands. You are not totally alone, but neither are you in the mainstream of vibrant life.

Did You Know?

Thirty percent of those diagnosed are children.

source: cureepilepsy.org/ aboutepilepsy/facts.asp

Hindrances coming out of the water and onto the beach are multi-dimensional. You may fear rejection of those on the beach . . . that you will not fit into the group(s) you wish to be a part of. You may feel inadequate to "play with the big boys." The water may have become so familiar to you, that coming out of the water makes you feel like "a fish out of water." But, it's also entirely possible that you get such great joy and fulfillment from the interior parts of your soul when you are alone in the water, that you feel no need to be on the beach, except for special times with your family or with particular persons. In essence, you have discovered that living underwater has become a productive and vibrant place to live; you have discovered that your ocean is teeming with meaningful life.

7

Sandwiches

The word *heal* comes from the Old English *haelan* and means not simply "to cure" but "to make whole."[20] —Norman Doidge, MD

The brain is a marvelously dynamic and ever-changing organ. My brain was thrilled with new stimulation, and when balanced with an adequate amount of sleep, it was capable of miraculous healing.[21] —Jill Bolte Taylor, PhD

Moods can change quickly.

Let's go back to six months after my illness. I felt excited about finally being considered seizure-free and being given permission to drive again. I felt energetic, like a teenager getting my first license. I felt ambitious, like a kid at Christmas. I felt respected as an actual adult again. I felt I was improving, similar to when I was released from the hospital.

I felt free.

This time, I didn't steal the keys and drive without permission. This time, I knew where to go and what to do. This time, I was in control.

I drove to the sandwich shop and parked in a clear place that would be easy for my limited memory to recall. I walked through the door and in the restaurant—then began shaking. Not because the line was long or the temperature inside was cold. I suddenly felt out of control. I was afraid. I knew I would not be able to place an order.

---

20 *The Brain's Way of Healing*, xx.
21 *My Stroke of Insight*, 117.

The first official order I'm placing post-illness, and I couldn't adjust to the stress. Panic attacks had not been part of my life before.

I stood, staring at the line of people ordering lunch. I looked at the menu and could read none of the words. Reaching for my keys, I wanted to leave.

But I didn't.

This was my chance to come ashore. To resist reluctance. To fight though the powerful current of fear and doubt. To push through by choice.

I got in the line, putting my shaking hands in my pockets.

The line was slowly moving toward the front, and my tension continued to grow. I was sweating.

Again, I considered leaving. Maybe it was too soon for my solo attempt. I would have many more chances.

The words on the menu seemed to be in a language I didn't know.

The people all around me looked like fictional characters in a movie like "The Truman Show." I was the only one not fitting in. They sat at tables eating, acting as if ordering lunch was a normal task. They engaged in dialogue with calmness and confidence, two traits I'd recently lost.

I was near the front of the line.

It was almost my time to order. This should be simple.

Pre-illness and post-illness Chris have this in common: no surprises related to food—order what you like; get the same thing each time; don't risk disappointment.

Did You Know?

Epilepsy can develop at any age and can be a result of genetics, stroke, head injury, and many other factors.

source: cureepilepsy.org/ aboutepilepsy/facts.asp

But nothing felt common this time.

With only one person in front of me, I had fifteen seconds to depart. No one would know why.

But I would.

I always would.

So sensing help from a greater power and stubbornness from a man who hated to lose, I stayed.

They asked for my order.

Without realizing I was remembering, I placed my order. Without looking at the menu I couldn't quite read or the food I might request incorrectly, I placed my order.

Underwater, I came ashore.

I laugh now each time I eat in a sandwich shop. I still order the same sandwich the same way. I request my full order as if all ingredients were turned into one word I might remember: six-inch turkey on wheat with lettuce, tomatoes, pickles, oil and oregano, with plain chips and a water.

How did I remember? Why is such a small thing to others such a huge thing to me?

I can't remember if I ordered to eat in or to go. I can't remember if I enjoyed the meal. I can't remember what else I did that day. But I remember embracing the tension. I recalled what fear and panic and desire to escape feel like. Maybe all those prayers for me had worked a little, but it took fighting through my fears to experience the answers.

Driving was fun again. Not habitual actions anymore, but a pleasure. Not always fun for those riding with me or those at home waiting, but a joy for me. Would I stop when I should? Would I remember directions? Would I arrive home?

Holding the steering wheel was one of many things I had taken for granted before plummeting underwater. I knew street names and busy times of day. I knew the best routes to life's important places like restaurants for breakfast and lunch and dinner, ballparks for baseball games with our sons, courts for basketball games with our sons, the office, the library, the theme parks, the beach, and home. I remembered how to get home. And my doctor's offices. I remembered how to get there.

All the knowing and remembering and driving and turning felt different now. My eyes could see a location that looked right and felt right. My mind seemed to process in slow motion no matter what speed the car was riding. Should I turn? Is this the place? I knew the answers—didn't I? The more I tried to think, the less successful the thinking seemed to be.

I could give more details but this is enough—just one reminder of many struggles to remember. I drove back to the hospital where I had almost died. I parked. There was no rush; I had an hour before my next appointment. I looked at directions and worked to memorize the five streets I would travel on. The people I needed to visit would be there waiting—they needed someone to talk to.

I left the car, walked into the hospital, and revisited the room where I almost died. A few minutes to reflect and process again. This me. This new me.

After speaking to a few friends in the hospital, I returned to the car. I cranked the engine and began rehearsing directions to my next location. I would remember the way there even if I forgot the street names. But I wanted to recall. I didn't want a few nouns to run away, hiding in portions of my brain.

They did, though. They hid.

And I could not find my way there. I drove, lost. Lost at the sea of familiar streets, of common roads, of recognizable intersections. Underwater. Unknowing. Unable to find my way.

Again, my mood changed quickly.

I had to call for help.

A practice that would become my new method of survival on the ocean of forgetfulness—calling for help.

Many people are reluctant to do that. We want to know and remember. Independence is our identity. We feel like we are losing that when we confess, "I don't remember," or ask, "Can you remind me?" or admit, "I forgot."

People encountering Alzheimer's or dementia or PTSD or TBI or many other health issues know about forgetting—unless their conditions have advanced to the canal of not realizing or remembering their forgetfulness.

Thinking of this and writing about it makes me want to hit save and leave the computer. I just want a sandwich.

But I choose to stay in the water of remembering.

I want you to stay here with me.

One of the many who helped keep our offices functioning during my illness and recovery was Dianne Chambers. She says my toughest challenges were my inability to recall names. "You could remember every detail of every conversation you ever had with or about someone," she said. "But you could not recall their name."

She knew there was more. "Controlling your emotions was another big challenge for you," she said. What about for her and others who worked with me? What about my family and friends? "It was very frustrating and heartbreaking for those of us who loved you, to watch you struggle to recall a word, a name, to know when to let you struggle and when to jump in and help you. As discreetly as possible, of course!"

Is there any positive in the new me, the-panic-attack-while-placing-a-lunch-order me, the forget-my-way-to-a-familiar-place me? Dianne said, "You had more patience, more tolerance with people. You became more approachable."

That is her thought about a positive memory. Comments from friends and caregivers are important. But the thoughts and comments swirling through our own minds define us and defeat us.

Or inspire us to ride the waves in this new life.

However the minds work. However the moods change. However the memories hide.

What's Helped Me

· Find other ways to exercise the brain. Seek to remember and repeat. Take tests. Listen to statements you hear on TV or radio or online and try to repeat each word. Try to memorize portions of songs, books, poems, quotes, and stories. And remember: refuse to get down on yourself when you don't do well. This is working and helping the brain, not testing or condemning the brain.

Chris Maxwell

8

Senses

Dostoevsky's seizures occurred periodically, every few months or days. Each one started with an ecstatic feeling which he could not fully describe.[22] —Eve LaPlante

What he saw was blue waves flecked with foam, and paler blue sky, both spreading without a break to the horizon.[23] —C.S. Lewis

"I don't understand."

She stated that sentence after listening to my story. As a college student studying to pursue a career in counseling, she wanted to hear my narrative about my illness and my life with epilepsy. She wanted to understand better—moving from books and theory to a face, to a personal story of pain, to application. So I told her of the days and the nights, the forgetting, the fears, the hoping, and the reality. I told her how I think and forget, how I become so exhausted as the brain works desperately to work correctly, how I wonder when a seizure might occur, and how I labor to find hope in the storm. I told her about writing with a rhythmic flow, motioning with a current of water where mental tide is crucial.

She listened well, proving she's probably pursuing the right career.

But that was her response: "I don't understand."

I waited a moment, allowing the silence a place in our conversation. The noise maker continued its rhythm, prohibiting those in nearby rooms from

---

22 *Seized*, 37.
23 C.S. Lewis, *The Voyage of the Dawn Treader*, The Chronicles of Narnia (New York: Harper Collins, 1952) 12.

hearing confessions in a counseling center. The sound of a bus driving by caused us both to glance out the window. A door in the room beside my office was opened then closed. Someone in the parking lot tapped to unlock their car.

I wanted to say, "I don't understand either."

Instead, I asked, "What do you not understand?"

I didn't know how she would answer. Did I not explain my situation adequately? Did I over complicate or over simplify? Did my brain fail in an effort to tell a story?

She looked out the window again, then down toward her feet, then slowly stared directly at me. She reached for tissues.

"I don't understand why anyone would have to go through this."

Understanding fully isn't required for life underwater.

Knowledge is important in grasping facts better. Research has been crucial to my own recovery. I've hunted information about encephalitis. I've chased data about epilepsy. I've pursued details about anti-epileptic medication, side-effects, speech therapy, brain chatter, neuroplasticity, and laughter.

> **What's Helped Me**
>
> • Keep sunglasses nearby if you are sensitive to lighting.
> • Watch the sun rise.
> • Watch the sun set.
> • Begin each day with a time of reflection. Set a few goals.
>
> **Chris Maxwell**

Pursuit of information provides results for what and how and when.

Not why.

There is really no answer to that question.

We can know what officially caused certain diseases and disabilities. Many we can't. We can often know the details. But not the why.

And a big step for me was becoming okay with that. Becoming okay with not knowing, with not understanding. To me, that isn't a desired outcome. It is life underwater.

A life I decided to embrace.

A life I recently decided to get to know even better.

Last year was my year of more tests. It had been ten years since my last MRI and EEG. I had not felt well—vision issues not caused by needing glasses, exhaustion not caused by working out, forgetfulness more than my usual amount, aura, stares, numbness, etc. My neurologist suggested it was time. I agreed.

I had the MRI that I wrote about in a previous chapter—I just don't remember which one.

I had an EEG that I'll write about at the end—if I remember.

We saw no new damage, adjusted medication slightly, and considered all would be okay. It was. But that made me think. My okay was no longer okay for me.

So my neurologist and I discussed other options. We set up an appointment for me to see a neuropsychologist.

Did You Know?

For many soldiers, suffering traumatic brain injury on the battlefield, epilepsy will be a long-term consequence.

source: cureepilepsy.org/ aboutepilepsy/facts.asp

Right after my illness, I wasn't capable of grasping life underwater. Now, I believed I was. I wanted all the information—no matter how bad—to reveal my true self to myself.

And that is what happened.

I sat in the office for the first meeting. We talked about my story, my condition, and my reason for being willing to be tested twenty years after the illness.

We discussed the plans—my next appointment would be a full day of mental testing, and the final appointment would be an evaluation of the test results. I didn't smile. Neither did the clinical health psychologist.

Those of you who know me know I would rather write about the sunrise I saw early that morning of my testing or about the moon smiling at the hotel window the night before. I would rather write about the full day of testing itself—the tension of searching through my brain in a brief amount of time to find words concealed, the pressure of sitting and staring and listening and trying so hard to remember, the weight of knowing I was not answering questions correctly, the strain of feeling like a little kid who would not pass my wife's test in her fourth-grade class. I would rather write about my turkey sandwich at my brief lunch break. I would rather write about the time I quickly stood out of frustration, and the one giving my test almost panicked as he tried so hard to keep his psychologist-in-training demeanor.

But I'll move on toward the results from my testing. I can understand parts of the document—enough to know about my weaknesses.

The opening lines seemed appropriate: *Punctual. Alert and oriented to person, location, and circumstances. Speech was within normal limits for volume, rate, and vocabulary. Thought process was logical, linear, and goal-oriented.*

Not bad. So far, I like their psychological gossip about me. But, like me, their observations began shifting: *The patient was observed to ask for repetition of test instructions on some subtests. On those occasions, he restated the instructions in his own words to ensure comprehension. He stated, "That's what I have to do to make sure I've got it."*

I want to restate three of their words: "on those occasions." Those of us with epilepsy or other similar conditions know about life "on those occasions." Restating to ensure comprehension? Yes, that is my life underwater. Repetition, rephrasing, restating: this adventure of remember and reinforce and recall. I'm astonished not everyone needs those responses "on those occasions."

Anyway, let's read on in this revelation of myself—the man who now has a new name, *The Patient: The patient applied systematic approaches to most testing tasks and utilized effective strategies in order to maximize performance (e.g., using a finger to track his location on a page, work the edges of a puzzle before filling the center, etc.). He demonstrated episodic frustration with testing, particularly on tasks he found challenging. He stated, "This is what I'm talking about" and on multiple occasions asked the administrator, "Wouldn't you be upset with this?"*

The one providing my test did not answer my question. I assumed he would be upset, and I felt a little more upset that he provided only the required stare—I wanted a heart.

Actually, during my lunch break, feeling like a child struggling to answer elementary questions but still being offered a brief recess, I could hear the voice from "The Wizard of Oz": "If I only had a brain." I could hear it in my head, my scarred head, my head being tested for seven hours with lunch on my own.

But let's go back to some of their comments. Systematic approaches? Yes, my method of helping myself remember, my labor of learning, my effort to feel a little like the more normal thinkers. Episodic frustration? That first word is not on my usable vocabulary, but I can guess its meaning. I don't disagree; I don't have to like it, though.

Who wouldn't be upset taking tests they could answer years before? Wouldn't something be more wrong with me if I didn't care? Sorry. I know you're not my therapist. I'm just revealing a little of my self-talk to you.

The patient asked for and was granted permission to stand during some of the tests' procedures. He was provided a break for lunch midway through the testing battery and did not ask for any additional breaks.

Reading those closing lines causes me to smile. They granted me permission to stand. I remember standing and seeing the facial expression of the man giving me the test. He said, "Are you okay?" Maybe he thought I was having a seizure. I wasn't. I needed to come ashore for a moment to think, to compete, to readjust.

Let's read on to their "Summary of Findings"—well, some of their "Summary of Findings."

- *He scored in the average range on measures of abstract verbal reasoning and vocabulary.*
- *Mild impairment was noted on a measure of required verbal information.*
- *Confrontation naming was in the severe impairment range.*
- *Working memory scores in this domain varied from the low average to superior average*
- *Processing speed scores on measures of processing speed were generally faster than the average individual.*
- *He demonstrated average ability on a measure of numeric sequencing.*
- *Performance was in the above average range of a measure of visual scanning and high average range on a measure of digit coding.*

I should probably stop here. The scores do not get better.

But I'll continue revealing more of the investigation about my ability, or inability, to remember.

- *He was able to recall ten elements from a narrative following a delay, resulting in mildly impaired performance.*

- *He was unable to recall any words from the word list non-contextual memory following either long or short delays and even with the aid of cues.*

- *Mr. Maxwell is highly attuned to cognitive difficulties he may experience and is strongly impacted by his perception of difficulties.*

- *Because of the changes notable from baseline functioning, the patient experiences initial frustration.*

- *To this point, the patient has not yet found a clear understanding to the nature and extent of his difficulties and, likewise, a prognosis.*

- *The patient has implemented an extensive set of compensatory strategies to accommodate his relative difficulties and has done so with success.*

- *Writing is an intensive process that necessitates left and right hemisphere, as well as frontal lobe involvement.*

What's Helped Me

· Hit pause in the middle of each day. Breathe deeply. Reflect and realize: even through the pain and difficulties, you are here and you are important.

Chris Maxwell

- *Continuing to engage these complex neurological networks is important in cognitive maintenance.*

- *Performance can be enhanced with reliance on feelings of familiarity (as opposed to recollection based mechanisms).*

- *Test results are indicative of both cognitive strengths as well as weaknesses. Strengths include frontal lobe functioning. Including processing speed, cognitive flexibility, working memory, and other aspects of executive functioning. His cognitive reserve in these areas served to compensate for deficits in other areas of cognition.*

At the airport, they ask for my driver's license or passport. To enter some offices, I just need an ID card. I can pay for a turkey sandwich or chocolate-chip-cookie-dough ice cream or a salad or new book with a card.

Who needs all that information about memory impairment, behavior abnormalities, left and right hemisphere, processing speed, neurological networks, or cognitive difficulties?

I do.

I want to know more about remembering less. I want to know what to do to improve.

Even if I can do nothing, I can be okay.

Even if I don't understand, I can let that make sense to me.

9

Smiles

There was a magic about the sea. People were drawn to it.
People wanted to love by it, swim in it, play in it, look at it.
It was a living thing that was as unpredictable as a great stage
actor: it could be calm and welcoming one moment, opening
its arms to embrace its audience, but then could explode
with its stormy tempers, flinging people around, wanting
them out, attacking coastlines, breaking down islands. It
had a playful side too, as it enjoyed the crowd, tossed the
children about, tipped over windsurfers, and occasionally
gave sailors helping hands—all done with a secret chuckle.[24]
—Cecelia Ahern

After years of fighting, I accepted that epilepsy is beyond my
control. . . . Whatever I don't know is OK. My life is OK.
I embraced that uncertainty and relished the surprises that
came with each day.[25] —Kristin Seaborg, MD

I was warned.

Those planning the event told me not to take it personally.

Before they explained the details, I was already starting to take it personally.

They informed me of the nation's reluctance to discuss epilepsy. Fathers
refused to allow their children to admit they lived with it. Caregivers showed

---

24 Cecelia Ahern, *The Gift* (New York: HarperCollins, 2009) 247.
25 *The Sacred Disease*, 173.

care through denial rather than help. Patients knew very little. The medical field struggled to offer help to patients who were never allowed to publicly "dive in" to the epilepsy adventure.

They told me my talk was first on the agenda. That was good. My brain and body were still living in the PM when Japan was already in tomorrow's AM. The sooner I could tell my story, the better.

Then they told me what I should not "take personally." As I talked in English and the audience could hear the translations coming almost at the same time in their own language, I was free to tell my story. A little slower pace than my typical tempo, but I was free to tell my story. But at the end, when the set scheduled twenty minutes of question and answer, I should expect little if any response. Maybe one would bow and honor me, but no one else would ask questions or voice their opinions. That was what I shouldn't take personally. It was cultural—not my failure to arouse interest. I was told to bow in return, to show respect, then move on to my seat. No one would ask questions, and the event could move on.

> **Did You Know?**
>
> In two-thirds of patients diagnosed with epilepsy, the cause is unknown.
>
> source: cureepilepsy.org/aboutepilepsy/facts.asp

That advice was helpful.

The prediction was incorrect.

I told my story. They listened. At the end, the expected leader bowed and nodded and talked to me in Japanese as my ears could hear it in English. But then something happened. Before I left the stage, others began to stand. Not sure what instigated the responses, but eyes opened and hearts cared. They talked. They asked questions. The company was voicing a desire to do more than sell products. They hoped to find a way to shift their culture's view about epilepsy.

At the end, when we completed the twenty-minute Q & A slot, I saw smiles. Not at me, really. Not at my telling of my own story. But smiles—that common revelation in any language—about believing the future of epilepsy can be different than its past. Smiles of promise and ambition. Smiles of a pledge and an oath. Smiles that did not need an interpretation.

They all began to take it personally in a different way. I call it ownership. They began taking personal responsibility to change how a culture and a world see epilepsy.

My evening at the banquet was breathtaking. I learned of their culture's music, dance, forms of art, and food. Through my interpreter, they learned more of my story through personal conversations. And I learned more of their stories—their wounds, their concerns, their lives underwater.

I looked at my friend Tom Roberts. All we could do was smile.

I recently smiled as I walked into a conference room the night before speaking there at a convention. That is best for me—knowing the environment early, rehearsing my way to the rooms, practicing the travel time, adjusting to the atmosphere.

Standing near the stage, I glanced toward the side. These four red letters trapped in a rectangle spelled one word that is common to most of us: EXIT.

I smiled. The next day I would be speaking to people who knew about hurt—some who have lived their underwater battle always seeking an escape. Their busyness or denial or addictions or obsessions or depressions are all related—they seek an exit.

One of the talks the following day would be about suicide and the unexpected deaths of those living with epilepsy. I would follow that with a story of hope. Now I knew how to place a bridge between the talks. We could all glance at the four letters we think and feel and consider: EXIT. But we can also smile as we choose to stay in the water, to stay the course, to stay in the voyage.

Desires to depart must not control us.

A future of hope and help and ambition can motivate us to exit our escape tendencies and endure our adventure.

While many epilepsy survivors live in cultures where there's still a negative stigma, more societies are changing. Not enough, but more are. In those environments, those with epilepsy struggle to admit when they have seizures or even confess their conditions. They're trained—intentionally in some places, unintentionally in others—to deny reality. To at least keep it silent or only among family. They're accused of demon possession, cultural embarrassment, and family shame. They're given no hope for the future and no help in the present.

But in many environments, those victims are welcomed. When we're given acceptance in their condition and permission to tell our stories, we're ready to grab the mic and talk for hours. We want to tell you our names as a way of defeating the stigma, of redefining ourselves and this life underwater. We want to take a breath, climb on your ship, and let all the passengers know what our adventure really feels like. We want to be understood and accepted. We want empathy. Confession, we guess, really is good for the soul. And our brains.

Caregivers are more cautious. Why? Notice the title they're listed as: caregivers. They care and they give. They give care.

They don't want to offend, to scare, to frighten, or to anger the one they care for. But, oh, the luggage they carry.

Researching advice for caregivers includes tips for helping those receiving care. What to do when the person has seizures. What to not do when the person has seizures. When to call 911 and when not to. What to say and what not to say. I want to see more advice about their own feelings of underwater.

What about those who face eating disorders, panic attacks, cancer, addictions, deception, anger, Parkinson's, Alzheimer's, depression? What about those who can't stop spending money or eating or lying? What about those who can't begin hoping or resting or laughing? What about those who can't imagine a day without hate or a day without pain?

I've been lost in the mall (maybe that is why I hate them, or maybe I don't like shopping, or maybe I hate spending money, or maybe the lights and sounds and environment aren't great for some of us, or maybe all of the above), at a ball game, on the road, and at an airport. I've been lost driving and walking and staring. But each time, I've found my way back. Or I have been found.

That is what I want for all of us. To find our way in the water. To find our way back to the shore. To find our way, to find ourselves, to find life. To find a true smile on our own faces.

But I know. It is not always simple.

To Tristin Johnson, a seizure felt "very sci-fi, like time freezing or crossing into another dimension." She said,

> In an instant, I am separate from the world as we know it. The hustle of everyday lives. The constant pace of morning to night. All still and silent. For a brief moment, my world

stands still. I am absorbed with fear and panic but also relieved of everyday rush. I am isolated from all that I know only to awaken and find that I've caught back up with time.

When we feel that way, notice the EXIT sign. Let's take a deep breath, choose to let the fears exit, and choose to keep ourselves where we belong.

We can also continue finding/seeking practical advice of what is best for us in our ocean of seizures and panic and another dimension.

Dr. Taylor remembers how "regaining vocabulary meant regaining some of the lost files in my brain. Just trying exhausted me, but slowly, word by hard-fought word, files were open, and I was re-introduced to the life of the woman I have been."[26] She reminds us what she needed most:

> **What's Helped Me**
>
> • End each day with a time of reflection. Evaluate your efforts to accomplish the goals. If you failed, forgive yourself, and plan ways to achieve those goals in the future.
>
> *Chris Maxwell*

- For successful recovery, it was important that we focus on my ability, not my disability.
- I needed people to celebrate the triumphs I made every day because my successes, no matter how small, inspired me.
- I made the cognitive choice to stay out of my own way during the process of recovery.
- I needed to welcome support, love, and help from others.
- My successful recovery was completely dependent on my ability to break down every task into smaller and simpler steps of action.
- I needed everyone to assume that I knew nothing so that I could relearn everything from the beginning.
- I needed my caregivers to teach me with patience.
- I needed people to come close and not be afraid of me.
- I needed my visitors to bring me their positive energy.[27]

26 *My Stroke of Insight*, 117.
27 Ibid, 117–120.

10

Stories

Epilepsy isn't a crime, but an illness. I'm not more or less of a person because I have seizures. . . . I was tired of hiding behind a veil of carefully constructed normalcy.[28] —Kristin Seaborg, MD

In 1888, in the south of France, a country doctor made a clever diagnosis. His patient was a thirty-five-year-old Dutch painter who had been living on the village of Arles for ten months. . . . On December 26, the doctor wrote in the patient's hospital chart, "M. van Gogh suffers from a form of epilepsy."[29] —Eve LaPlante

I tell a story about the swelling of my brain caused by encephalitis. I tell a story of always-healthy-Chris getting sick, of being in the ER and almost dying, of spending days in the hospital, of not remembering the names of our three sons, of a nurse coming to our house three times a day after I was finally released, of being a man who communicated for a living then needing months of speech therapy. I tell a story about resulting brain damage, severe scar tissue throughout that damaged brain especially in my left temporal lobe, change in personality, radical mood swings, and now living with long-term effects like epilepsy and short-term memory issues and the need to nap. I tell a story about me, the fit husband and dad and pastor and coach, becoming the very sick me who tried very hard to be the former me but couldn't do most of what he'd

---

28 *The Sacred Disease*, 210.
29 *Seized*, 1.

done before. I tell of forgetting names, forgetting events, forgetting how to spell, and forgetting something else, but I can't remember what. I tell of making things worse as I tried to make myself better. That's the story I tell.

That's the storm where the wind seems to still blow at times, the waves don't seem to ever fully calm at times, and the shore feels far, far away at times.

That's the story I tell—having trouble saying what I want to say. That's the story I live—as I reach for my meds, as I hold tightly to modern electronic devices that work to help my brain do its job a little better, as I stare while seeking a noun in my brain. That's the storm I feel around me, within me, surrounding me—when my story isn't sounding so fine to me.

> **What's Helped Me**
>
> • Notice your biggest fears. Seek help in learning from those fears and overcoming them.
>
> *Chris Maxwell*

Sorry if that phrase sounds childish to you. It is just the truth. I feel like a little kid in a not-so-young-man's body.

But my story is not the only one. There are so many stories. Real life stories. Narratives about life, symbolically, underwater. I want to introduce you to a few of my friends who have different, yet similar stories.

Here is Destiny's story—she is young and has faced so many disappointments:

My name is Destiny Burns. I'm twenty years old. I have intractable versions of both generalized and partial epilepsy with five different forms of seizures. I was born with it and had both absence and myoclonic seizures as a child, but was not diagnosed until age thirteen when I had a generalized tonic-clonic seizure. We then found out that I had epilepsy, but at that point, had no idea how much it was going to impact my life down the road. There, for the first year or so after diagnosis, it wasn't so bad. I had a seizure maybe every month or so and was able to live a kind of normal life. But then all of a sudden, everything changed.

By age seventeen, I was having too many smaller seizures daily to even attempt to count, and it started to take its toll on me. Over time, it has continued to get worse and worse. I have tried every anti-convulsant medication for my types of seizures, with no success of seizure control. At nineteen, I was implanted with a Vagus Nerve Stimulator in my left chest area which sends electrical signals to my brain at a regular pace—similar to a heart pacemaker. Now, at age twenty, my seizures are still considered "uncontrollable" by my epilepsy specialist. At this point in time, I average sixty or more seizures daily of mixed types.

Epilepsy has been very stressful and hard for me to deal with growing up. I have always been that person off to the side from the others my age, not able to drive or go to concerts or participate in any activities that might trigger me to seize, not being able to go anywhere unless someone was with me who knew how to take care of me. I wish people in this world understood how hard it is for people like me, feeling so unaccepted by society and like we have to hide our condition from the world in order to be treated like we are even human.

Did You Know?

In over 30 percent of patients, seizures cannot be controlled with treatment.

source: cureepilepsy.org/ aboutepilepsy/facts.asp

Epilepsy has so many frustrations that come along with it, like having all of the paramedics in the area know me by name, as well as all of the staff at the hospital emergency room. All of the bruises and scars, all of the marks left on my arms from being stuck for IVs, walking around looking like a pin-cushion, all of the times I am embarrassed because I forget things so much: it's my normal. I've been injured so many times by my seizures that I often refrain from doing things I want to do for fear of being hurt. I have been burnt so badly from seizing while trying to cook food for myself or just by having a seizure while taking a shower that I have had to have skin surgeries. I wake up in the floor of the shower with water spraying me in the face and automatically know what happened. I wake up surrounded by strangers at a grocery store telling me "ma'am, it's okay, lie still, the ambulance is on its way . . ." even though I don't need paramedics, but there's no way to express to people that this is the normal for me.

This is my life. I live it every day, but it's something I've had to learn to cope with. I know inside that this will never go away, this is a lifelong battle for me, but I still pray that one day I will wake up a different person, one who is normal. I push through, day in and day out, and try to live my life to the best of my abilities, using my talents in music and art to help me along the way. I may not be able to work or drive, but I can do other things, and as long as I am able to do that, I will.

Epilepsy is part of me, but it is not me.

I met Jeff Klauk at an epilepsy event. After he told me his name, I did what I have to do: I wrote it down. I also did what I like to do: I researched him. I'm not a golfer, but I love sports. Jeff is a golfer who is now learning about life underwater—life with epilepsy:

My journey with epilepsy started in June 2006 at a Web. com Tour professional golf event in Knoxville, Tennessee. I was tied for fifteenth entering the weekend when I had a tonic-clonic seizure and was forced to withdraw from the tournament. One out of twenty-six of us will develop epilepsy (multiple unprovoked seizures) in our lifetime. So when I had my second seizure about two months later at another Web. com event, it was time to seek treatment. I began seeing a neurologist here in Jacksonville, Florida, and tried lots of different medications. Finally, I was able to get my tonic-clonic seizures under control. After being diagnosed with epilepsy, purple, the color of epilepsy, became one of my favorite colors.

In 2008, with my seizures under control, I was able to accomplish a dream of earning my PGA Tour card by finishing third on the Web.com money list. Playing on the PGA Tour in 2009 was fantastic, and my game was great. I had three, fourth-place finishes and was able to fulfill a lifelong dream by playing in The Players Championship. I grew up playing the TPC Sawgrass course as my dad, Fred, was the golf course superintendent.

On December 24, 2010, I started having another type of seizure called complex partial seizures. They last one to two minutes, and you lose consciousness for a short period. I would generally pop right back, feeling okay but wondering what just happened.

No medicine was controlling my complex partial seizures, so in 2012, I decided to have brain surgery at Emory University Hospital in Atlanta. I hoped the doctors would locate the area of my brain where my seizures were coming and remove that area. I was in the hospital for twenty-three days, but they weren't able to precisely determine the area where the seizures were originating. However, after trying several medications, I finally found a medicine that helped control my seizures.

But even when you think things are improved with controlling your seizures, it can change the next day. In August 2016, I had a break-through seizure again. So it's back to no driving until I can be seizure free for six months. I can't thank all my family and friends enough for their support and help through the years. Battling any problem is all about the support you have, and I'm so fortunate to have my parents, my wife Shanna's family, and a countless number of friends nearby.

I recently transitioned from a sixteen-year professional playing career to a role with Perfect Golf Event as the Manager of Tournaments and events for the new digital platform designed for charitable and sponsored golf tournament organizers. This would enable them to raise more money for their causes.

Having played in many pro-ams through the years as a professional, I know how important fundraising events are for individual and corporate causes. Since I have epilepsy and want to help raise funds for the Epilepsy Foundation and other causes, I understand how vital it is to be prepared for events so that organizations can raise the most money for their charitable initiative. There is a growing demand for this kind of service, and being involved with Perfect Golf Event is intriguing because it allows me to stay involved in golf and help others.

Mary Ann Heinsohn knows about epilepsy and seizures and medications. She also knows this life underwater can become more literal than figurative:

It was a morning just like so many others. Feeling tired and exhausted, all I wanted to do was just shut my eyes; but, too much was on my plate. A friend would soon be arriving to sit for my mother. I had to redeem the free time and just keep moving.

Driving out of my neighborhood, I literally "lost it!" For one brief moment, I "zoned out" and entered the world of epilepsy. Little did I realize, I had exited my gated community, crossing four lanes of traffic, and missing phone poles and trees. When the fog in my brain lifted, I looked outside my window only to see the vegetation surrounding my car, and the spectators watching my every move. Water was slowly creeping up from the floor. Without one ounce of fear, I kicked out the passenger window knowing that time was of the essence, and watched the water as it began to pour in.

> ### What's Helped Me
>
> · Notice your deepest worries. Learn what causes those worries but refuse to be controlled by them.
>
> *Chris Maxwell*

As I swam to the bank, EMS extended their hand to help me to dry land. When they asked if I wanted to go to the hospital, my response was, "No. I have epilepsy. There's nothing a hospital can do for me. You see, sir, I'm losing my mother to ovarian cancer. Acting as her primary caregiver placed undue stress on my life, which provoked this seizure. If you could just return me to my home to get out of these wet clothes, I would be most appreciative."

Kristy Rastle has a nice laugh. But her life hasn't always been full of laughter. She also knows about the pains from life with epilepsy:

Flash: A searing pain in my wrist from medication being pushed through my vein. Flash: A nurse sticking her head into the room and 'hushing' a growing group of friends who were laughing too loudly. Flash: Seeing the multi-colored and braided Muppet hair of a close friend with the bright lights of the hospital room above her. Flash: At home now and throwing up tomato soup. That's all I remember from the first day of the new me, in all about ten seconds.

The next two weeks I spent in a haze—unable to think, not really able to speak due to a badly bitten tongue, and slowly realizing that the hour-long tonic-clonic seizure I had that day had taken about half of the memories I had collected throughout my life, including the information I needed to do my job. A visit to a neurologist and a few tests confirmed the unimaginable to me, that I now had epilepsy—with three different seizure types.

My journey, now seventy years later has been one of piecing together what was lost (which comes back in flashes), while also creating something new. There have been soaring highs as I discover the new me, but as the seizures continue unabated even with many, many different treatments, also periods of absolute soul-crushing lows, I find strength now in not only conquering my limitations, but also accepting them. I can never go back to the person I was before epilepsy, but I can be something different, something unexpected.

Did You Know?

Uncontrolled seizures may lead to brain damage and death.

source: cureepilepsy.org/ aboutepilepsy/facts.asp

11

Seasons

You have brains in your head.
You have feet in your shoes.
You can steer yourself
any direction you choose.[30] —Dr. Seuss

Crisis doesn't make a person. It reveals you for what you
are. You don't know who someone is until adversity comes.
It shows the cracks, and the cracks are where God leaks
through.[31] —Leonard Sweet

My friend Lakeisha has offered a new medication that's helped many of us:
her laughter. In our meetings, texts, meals, and phone calls, she helps herself
and her friends survive in our underwater escapades. She laughs. It spreads. I
once started laughing after hearing her laugh but I had no idea why she was
laughing.

Not all of her adventures underwater have been comical. But through the
pain, she has found a way to see it all through a better perspective. Here is the
letter Lakeisha wrote to her old self:

Dear LaKeisha,

I know what you are going through is tough. You didn't
see this coming! At twenty-two years old, at the peak of your
career, you had a beautiful baby girl and you owned your first
home. You worked so hard to get where you are. You've been

---

30 Dr. Seuss, *Oh, the Places You'll Go!* (New York: Random House, 1990) 2.
31 Leonard Sweet, *Summoned to Lead* (Grand Rapids, MI: Zondervan, 2004),
    96.

a shoulder to lean on for many people. The morning you left to help your godmother in her time of need, you never thought that your own life would forever change. When this journey first began, your mother gained her wings and soon your brother followed. But you were okay with that because your faith kept you persevering, and your daughter was always your strength.

But your life started to change one night before you got ready for the night shift at work. Your daughter, Gabrielle, wanted tacos because, let's be honest, your cooking was never really that great, and that's all you knew how to cook. So off you went to the store to get the ingredients. But you found yourself home a few hours later not sure how you drove there and back. You were scared. You didn't know what happened. You called your job to tell them you weren't coming in. Underneath your pounding headache and tears of worry, you could see the fear in your daughter's eyes. She was scared to come near you! I know you wondered why because you're her mom, not some monster or stranger.

> **Did You Know?**
>
> Up to 50,000 Americans die each year from seizures and related causes.
>
> source: cureepilepsy.org/aboutepilepsy/facts.asp

LaKeisha, it wasn't easy going into the emergency room that night, but you wanted to know what happened. You had always been healthy, so this was all new to you. They told you that you possibly had a seizure. Possibly, were they not sure? You left even more confused. There was some sense of relief because at least it had a name. But you still had questions like, How many more am I going to have?

Why did I have it? How is this going to affect me? You were also in denial. You had been through enough in life already: adoption, teen mom, single parent, losing family. You had endured all of those trials. Was this your final test? When you followed up with your PCP, he determined that, based on your daughter's description of what happened, it was a seizure. You saw your first neurologist. You believed he would hold not only the key to all of your questions but that he would hold the cure to this "seizure thing," and that you would pass yet another one of life's tests.

Your father came with you to see the first neurologist, which made you feel calm that morning. The appointment was quick: they ran tests and set up another appointment for you to have more tests done. Over the span of six weeks, you had MRIs and EEGs, and everything looked normal. But for you, it wasn't. The doctor didn't seem to be hearing your complaints of headaches, déjà vus, and even having another seizure. He just gave you more pills. He told you it's just a seizure disorder and that you should go back to work. You didn't go to school for medicine, so you wholeheartedly trusted what he said. But deep down inside, you knew something wasn't right.

After being off of work following a seizure that you had six months prior, you were okay to go to work. So you left downtown Chicago and went to fill up your gas tank. You kept thinking to yourself that morning that something just wasn't right. You pumped your gas, and the next thing you remember you awoke to being questioned by a sheriff in the back of an ambulance. What happened? You kept calling your daughter's name out because you thought she was in the car. You had been on your way to spend time with her before work. Between the sheriff's nonstop questioning—were you drinking, on drugs, or just sleepy—you could hear the EMT say to you, "Miss, you were in an accident. You had a seizure." He kept asking if you had epilepsy and you kept saying, "No, I have a seizure disorder." It was too much. Your fears were getting the best of you.

You were relieved that no one else was hurt. But inside, you begin to plead with God. You promised him that if he let you live, you would do better, stop and smell the roses, and help people in every way you could. LaKeisha, he kept his promise, and I see you keeping yours.

I know sitting in the hospital in the ICU was hard. Having eight broken ribs, two broken legs, two broken fingers, a broken hand, a broken ankle and three surgeries was not easy. Your road to recovery will be rocky because you've had to face your fears of trying to hold on to who you used to be. Don't worry about the house you lost, the job you lost, and the friends who left. One day, you'll realize this all had to happen to form who you will soon become. I know living in a shelter wasn't what you imagined either. Your father didn't understand why he couldn't fix this for his little girl, so he chose to tell people that your accident happened because you were driving too fast. This was his way of dealing with it. More so, I know it hurts that your trust in your physician was broken. How do you begin to repair that? So much has changed, LaKeisha, but I see a light up ahead, so you just hold on. The doctor on call in the ICU, who would later become your new neurologist, finally diagnosed you with epilepsy.

He was an angel that day. You were afraid, but he handled you with care. He taught you so much about seizures. You remember when you came in depressed one day to an appointment. You had tried your best to dress up. But he looked at you and said, "LaKeisha, how long have you been like this?" You burst in tears—tears of joy. Your doctor cared enough to notice a problem that you couldn't carefully articulate. He showed the same care when it was time to switch your medicines. You were scared at first, but he walked you through the process. He even helped you join a support group and get counseling for new patients. When you had a side effect you didn't like, he talked to you and taught you how to be an ambassador for your health.

Look at you now! You've moved out on your own to Atlanta with your favorite nieces and discovered life. Your seizures are less frequent, and your side effects are tolerable. Even when you became pregnant with your other children and you had to go on another AED, you were afraid at first. But you researched and took part in pregnancy registries.

Yes, I know insurance companies are tough to deal with, especially when you have epilepsy. But you follow up and make sure your doctor does their part by making sure that your insurance understands that your medications cannot be altered. You file paperwork and do appeals if needed. Medications are costly, but you've sacrificed your needs for them. You may not get to enjoy extra things, and it puts you on a tight budget, but your health is priority, and I applaud you for making that sacrifice.

I know being a police officer was your dream, and your ambition was to finish college. It had been your dream since you were seven years old to serve and protect others. I know your dream didn't become a reality because of epilepsy. But look at how far you've come. LaKeisha, you were in a wheelchair for almost three years. Now you wear your leg brace with style. Your family, friends, and people everywhere admire your strength. You didn't quit despite the odds that were stacked against you. Yes, being a mom of four children—Gabrielle nineteen; Gabriel nine; Grace seven; Gracelynn two—isn't easy. I know you're tired. It can be a challenge, but keep your head up. When you really take a step back and look at your life, you can see that your dream and ambition

> **What's Helped Me**
> · Allow yourself to cry.
> · Allow yourself to laugh.
> · Allow yourself to schedule times to rest the brain and the body.
> *Chris Maxwell*

weren't stopped. They were just merely deferred as you grew up to handle the *"new you"* and understand your life's purpose. You discovered self-love, and confidence in your abilities and yourself despite the circumstances.

See some people think the greatest tragedy is death, but I think that it's living this life and never living out your true purpose. Look at you now! You found your purpose. You may not be seizure free, and that's okay. But you went to college, and thanks to the UCB Epilepsy Family Scholarship, you finished college, not just with one degree, but two!

You've served people as a pastor, mentor, and an epilepsy advocate. And now as a confidence coach, you help people discover their life's purpose so no one else is ever left to feel alone on this life's journey. You give people hope because you are hope: Helping Others Past Epilepsy 2 Endure!

She gets it. Her self-talk reinforces positive beliefs. Her life, though underwater, is important. She is important. Her condition is not her only identity.

Go through her letter and think about yourself. Write a note to you. Challenge, dare, encourage, and inspire yourself.

Realize the season you are in. Accept it. Choose what you can do to live this season correctly.

Enjoy life underwater. Pursue abundant life in the water. And come ashore when it is time.

12

Survivors

There can be no real hope unless it somehow embraces, unashamedly, the presence of real suffering in the world. . . .[32]
—Mark Yaconelli

We do not become hopeful by talking about hope. We become hopeful by entering darkness and waiting for the light.[33]
—Mark Yaconelli

I have enjoyed my conversations with Heather Overton, and I love listening when she tells her story. She cares for people. Her story reminds us that being survivors gives us a chance to help others survive and thrive.

I have joked in the past that I feel like a "cat with nine lives," and you'll hear why as I tell my story.

My mother was sick, and in an effort to diagnose her, she had a number of X-rays. My brother was only five months old, so she didn't even consider she could be pregnant. When she realized she was, her internist suggested she have an abortion because the fetus probably suffered substantial damage that would lead to all kinds of birth defects. But my mother's obstetrician and the radiologist concurred that she did not receive enough radiation to harm the fetus and felt that the baby would be just fine. The internist wasn't happy with that decision.

---

32 Mark Yaconelli, *The Gift of Hard Things: Finding Grace in Unexpected Places* (Downers Grove, IL: InterVarsity Press, 2016,) 98, 99.
33 Ibid.

I was born a week early and very blue because the umbilical cord was wrapped around my neck. We don't know if this or the radiation is the cause for my seizures, but to this day, my parents have said that they never regretted their decision. They chose not to end my life. But my birth was the beginning of a long and challenging journey—but that's what life is, right?

When I was eighteen months old, my parents were picking me up at my baby-sitter and something unexpected happened. Instead of being greeted with my usual happy face, they were horrified when I suddenly gasped, my eyes rolled back into my head, and I went into convulsions. This was the beginning of a long path leading us to numerous neurologists in hopes of getting to the bottom of what was going on "inside my little head" (as they say). As a toddler, the initial diagnosis was febrile seizures. When I got older, they were categorized as absence seizures. I would experience staring spells, which my dad described as "the lights are on, but nobody's home." However, around age seven, my seizures seemed to stop. After being seizure-free for two years, the doctor slowly weaned me off all medication.

> **Did You Know?**
>
> The mortality rate among people with epilepsy is two to three times higher than the general population.
>
> *source: cureepilepsy.org/ aboutepilepsy/facts.asp*

During my freshman year in high school, I took keyboarding. I remember sitting in front of the computer with the piece of paper covering my hands and the keyboard so I couldn't peek. All of a sudden, I'd start having these jerks. There would be a jumble of letters on the computer screen, and I'd get so frustrated because we were being graded on our accuracy. To be honest, it scared the heck out of me, and I knew something was terribly wrong. After a couple of weeks of being yelled at by my teacher for "playing" around in class, I finally went home and told my parents that something was wrong.

I was diagnosed with JME or Juvenile Myoclonic Epilepsy. Since I had no recollection of my first diagnosis, I had a difficult time dealing with the fact I had epilepsy. There is no way to know for sure why the seizures returned, but the doctors have speculated that the massive hemorrhaging I experienced may have triggered their return. My neurologist was great and made me feel at ease, but he wasn't able to help relieve the seizures. We tried medication after medication and every combination possible, but nothing seemed to work. During all of this I was having multiple seizures at school. They called the paramedics for me at least once a month. Trying different medications all of the time made me sick, so I spent a lot of time in the nurse's office sleeping or vomiting. (Sounds lovely, doesn't it?) Although, my classmates and I had to laugh: it became a bit of a running joke at school that every time a squad was called, they inevitably knew they were coming for me. I fell down the stairs at school more times than I can count. I was lucky to have attended a small all-girl school with the friends I'd known all my school years. They were very understanding and supportive.

When I was seventeen, my cousin risked her own safety to make sure I was okay. Amber and I were talking on the phone when I started to gasp and dropped the phone. She knew that I was having a seizure and that no one else was home. So Amber, her brother, and her mom drove to my house. Amber stood on her brother's shoulders and he boosted her up onto the roof where she basically fell into my bedroom through the window. She told me that she didn't really think too much about her own safety, only that she wanted to make sure I didn't get hurt, fall down, or something even worse.

I was really disoriented, and they asked me all of the usual questions like, "What day is it?" I guess I argued about even having had a seizure. I think I was embarrassed or felt guilty that my family had to check on me. This made me angry, and

I'd deny that anything happened. Although my response at the time was not what you'd call "grateful," I am very grateful for Amber, not just for what she did that day, but all of the times she's been there for me as a caring cousin and my best friend.

By the time I was eighteen, my seizure activity had increased—I was experiencing three to four tonic-clonic seizures a week and hundreds of myoclonic seizures. I became so weak and terrified that I felt like giving up. I actually wanted to have brain surgery because I wanted a "cure" so badly, but nothing was working.

After I graduated from high school, I moved on to college. My parents worried about me going to college, but they knew how much value my independence and need to accomplish this. Although attending college full time was a great and new experience in my life, I was also around strangers who didn't understand epilepsy. This was my first experience with really having to educate others about the condition. I had a couple of seizures in class. Each time it happened, I went back to the next class and used the opportunity to educate my classmates and teachers about epilepsy and seizure first aid. I knew I needed to be open to questions and not be embarrassed about my condition. As hard as it could have been, putting a positive spin on the situation helped me get through it easier.

In March 2003, about a month after I started a job at the University of Nebraska at Omaha, I had a severe tonic-clonic seizure. The ambulance was called, and off I went to the hospital again. That evening, a resident attempted to do a spinal tap, and my heart stopped. The next thing I knew, I had about ten people over me saying "Heather, are you with me?" (This was my sixth near-death experience.) I continued to go to school and work full time, and I continued to have three to four seizures a week. I felt like my world was crashing down around me.

Overall, attending college wasn't easy. I had a few setbacks. In addition to my epilepsy, I also had two surgeries within two years, causing stress and increased seizure activity. This is when I used my cat lives numbers four and five. The first time I had my gall bladder removed, and another time, I had to have my appendix removed. The surgeries were followed by a bout with bronchial pneumonia. All of these health problems forced me to take three semesters off from school. It has been frustrating, but I was determined not to let epilepsy control me or hold me back. I am proud to now be a graduate!

Then everything changed when the Nebraska Medical Center opened the Epilepsy Center in 2003. I really liked my neurologist, but my parents convinced me to at least meet the epileptologist.

On my first visit, I was very demanding. I was angry my parents had made me go and so frustrated with everything I'd already been through. I guess I thought, "I've tried everything; how can you possibly help?" I told him that I wanted to continue to work and go to school full time. I wanted to drive. But most of all I really just wanted to be seizure free.

> **What's Helped Me**
> · Be quick to hear.
> · Be slow to talk.
> · Be slow to become angry.
>
> *Chris Maxwell*

The epileptologist sat in his chair and patiently listened, then said, "Honestly, we'll do the best we can." And together, we finally found the combination that worked for me. In time, I became seizure free. Now, I take five different medications in very precise dosages, keeping me seizure free for more than eight years. Your experience may be different from mine; that's why it's important to talk with your doctor to determine what's right for you.

I still experience some side effects like fatigue. There were also times I noticed that I had trouble concentrating and experienced mild depression, but I learned ways to combat these effects. To help me combat fatigue, I take naps, and I love naps. When I think back to kindergarten and how we begged them to skip naptime, I have to laugh and say, "What were we thinking?" Now, I have to admit, most days after work, I will take a "cat nap," and on weekends I am able to nap throughout the day. Yes, I do experience some side effects, but I find them manageable.

I can tell you it may have taken me and my family twenty years of education and perseverance to find me seizure freedom, but it was worth the wait. Part of my success has been my amazing epileptologist. Part of it has been my parents' "never give-up" attitude. Part of it was me being demanding. Don't give up, keep asking, and keep looking for the right treatment. My epileptologist really listened to what I wanted and helped me find a way to get there.

Did You Know?

Risk of sudden death among those with epilepsy is twenty-four times greater.

source: cureepilepsy.org/
aboutepilepsy/facts.asp

My family and I were so grateful, after so many years of frustration and dashed hope, we felt motivated to help other families living with epilepsy. So in April of 2004, with the support of the Nebraska Medical Center, my mother and I started the first Nebraska Epilepsy Support group.

The support group has given me a chance to see things from my family's perspective. I heard my mother tell me what it felt like to be the parent of a child struggling with epilepsy. I learned she cried all of the time as I was growing up and wished she'd had a support group to help listen and understand. My sister recently cried when she attended a meeting and, for the first time, understood how difficult it's been for me—just living day to day.

I encourage all people with all conditions to tell their stories and get the word out. Telling our stories, building awareness, and helping educate others helps us heal and learn from our own disabilities. Having epilepsy has helped to mold me into the person I am today, and I would never change the way my life has turned out.

No matter how challenging your situation may feel, don't give up hope. You need to be your own biggest advocate. Even if it seems like a lot of work, find an epileptologist who understands your needs and is willing to work with you because it is possible to find a medication or medications with tolerable side effects that work for you. You can take control of your epilepsy and take back your life. Who knows? Maybe you're more like me, and you'll have nine or so chances to try again. It's not so bad being compared to a cat; after all, they are also known for always "landing on their feet," right?

What part of Heather's story do you relate to? Who are the family members and friends who can help you pursue a better life with epilepsy? Why do you think so many people refuse to pursue help from new doctors and from family members? How can an epilepsy group provide encouragement?

13

Stains

Spend the afternoon, you can't take it with you.[34] —Annie Dillard

There is always an enormous temptation in all of life to diddle around making itsy-bitsy friends and meals and journeys for itsy-bitsy years on end. It is all so self-conscience, so apparently moral. . . . I won't have it. The world is wilder than that in all directions, more dangerous and bitter, more extravagant and bright. We are . . . raising tomatoes when we should be raising Cain, or Lazarus.[35] —Annie Dillard

I have enjoyed my conversations with Tim Tilt. He is friendly and kind, and I can see how he cares deeply for all people—especially those of us with epilepsy. Many of our soldiers live with these struggles. They need to hear his story. I love listening to it. I think you will too.

One morning in January of 1979, after a sleepless night with our five-month-old son, Aaron, I got up as quietly as possible and hopped on my motorcycle to ride the twenty-five miles to work. The last thing I remember was passing over Ackerman Road at about seventy miles an hour. What happened next—I guess I'll actually never know—but when I "came to," I was riding down the access road next to the freeway, barely fast enough to keep my balance.

---

34 Annie Dillard, *Pilgrim at Tinker Creek* (New York: HarperCollins, 1974) 274.
35 Ibid.

Thankfully, it was still early, and there was barely any traffic. I pulled over to the side of the road, shut the engine off, and sat there just staring into space, wondering what in the world was going on. I was confused, stark-raving terrified, but of what, I didn't know. I felt extremely depressed, almost ready to cry, and absolutely dead-tired.

But after that "incident," nothing happened that made me even want to talk about it, much less worry. Then one evening, around midnight in September of 1979, almost nine months after my experience on the motorcycle, it happened again. Thankfully, I was in my car. When I started to realize that something was wrong, I was barely idling down a poorly lit neighborhood street in an unfamiliar part of San Antonio. My chest and left shoulder were really sore, evidently from the shoulder strap of the seat belt. The car was thumping, bumping, and rattling along, making a horrible screeching sound, and it was extremely hard to steer. My front left tire was completely gone; its wheel smashed flat.

> **What's Helped Me**
>
> • Do not go to sleep angry. Find healthy ways (journaling, praying, seeing a counselor, etc.) of refusing to hold the anger inside or using it to attack someone.
>
> *Chris Maxwell*

I felt confused, scared to death, and was shaking like a leaf, and I barely made it back home. Monday morning, at the doctor's office, I met with a physician's assistant. When I finished telling him everything I could remember, he excused himself and got another lieutenant. By the time they were finished with me that morning, I had been called a liar, threatened with at least an article 15 (a form of non-judicial punishment) if not a court martial, and accused of doing drugs or driving while intoxicated. Yet, my test results showed absolutely nothing.

I was then admitted to Wilford Hall for a myriad of tests. It was kind of a familiar place for me because that's where our son was born. I figured that I'd be in pretty good hands. But the first several days I was treated like a criminal, even as they were running tests on me, including an EEG, sleep deprivation, a spinal tap, a neuropsychological exam, and others. Psychologists and psychiatrists had to know every detail and kept trying to get me to admit I was lying. They even had a chaplain come in and counsel me on the negative effects of living a lie.

In the end, after a long and exhausting series of tests, I was diagnosed as having temporal lobe seizures (epilepsy), and was started on a low dosage of medication to help control them. When the doctors sat me down and told me the diagnosis, it was—to say the least—a shock. Up until that time, I didn't even know that there was any kind of seizure but a tonic-clonic, and I sure didn't know anyone who had them. They told me "be careful, don't drive, don't do anything dangerous, and make sure you take your medication every day."

Did You Know?

Epilepsy results in an estimated annual cost of $15.5 billion in medical costs and lost or reduced earnings and production.

source: cureepilepsy.org/ aboutepilepsy/facts.asp

I felt fine, except for some mild depression, and, the following Monday, went back to work. Nothing seemed out of the ordinary, except that I couldn't drive.

The next two years in the Air Force were pretty non-eventful as far as my seizure disorder was concerned. I did have an occasional seizure, but they seemed to be under moderate control and only lasted about thirty seconds to a minute, instead of ten to fifteen minutes like the first two.

After I got out of the Air Force, I landed a job making custom furniture and doors. But unfortunately, my seizure activity began to noticeably increase. Usually they started with auras. I would feel nervous, scared almost to death of nothing in particular, and have odd smell and taste sensations—like something nauseatingly sweet.

Sometimes I just sit or stand and stare off into space, totally unaware of what's going on around me. Often, I'll be smacking and licking my lips. If I felt a seizure coming on at work, I'd shut off my equipment and make a mad dash to the bathroom. I had started driving again, but unfortunately, I had another auto accident—thankfully a minor one. The police told me to stop driving.

At work, the fact that I couldn't drive due to epilepsy was not a disability because once I got to work, I could do my assigned job. I was told it was my problem; if I didn't like it, I could quit. In fact, on more than one occasion, different supervisors—civilian and military—told me that they were hoping I would. I even had a high-ranking civilian say that a "spazmo" like me had absolutely no right doing what I did. That kind of comment was repeated by a lot of people, but I hunkered down and developed a tough outer layer. But on the inside, I was miserable.

Besides the fact I had a high-pressure job, the struggle with the personnel office and the negative treatment I was getting was taking its toll. My seizure activity sky-rocketed. The doctors caring for me at the VA Hospital were concerned, and in 1991, they convinced me to enter the hospital for a series of tests. But, after nineteen days, the results were inconclusive and did not indicate why my seizures were increasing in frequency. As the weeks, months, and years passed, the situation became difficult to bear. I called in sick more and more and was becoming very depressed.

Dark thoughts just wouldn't escape me.

Then, in August of 1998, I was among the first people at the VA hospital in San Antonio to have a Vagal Nerve Stimulator (VNS) implanted to help control my seizures. I did experience some favorable results, though it wasn't what I'd hoped for. I still felt down and depressed. It got to the point that I was so depressed that I just felt like, "what's the use of living?" Then, one day, a coworker launched into her usual cruel remarks about me and set me off. Since I'd been considering suicide for months, I already had a plan in mind, one of several actually.

I always carried a "special" bag which I secretly kept in my backpack. That little bag contained everything I needed to get the job done. But, there in the blackness and depths of despair, something clicked inside me. I suppose it was a moment of clarity. I pulled out my little bag, quickly handed it to a friend, and walked out without any explanation. I went through the high security front gate, dropped my badge on the counter, and left.

My employer, family, friends, relatives were absolutely shocked—everything from extreme concern about my well-being to absolute outrage that I had walked out of a great-paying job with great benefits. As a result, six months later, in April of 1999, I was medically retired. Because I took the right steps and got the help I so desperately needed—and deserved—I survived. I began my emotional recovery and regained my sense of well-being. And today, I'm really thankful for that—I really am.

After I started working again, my doctor and I decided to add a new medication to help control my seizures. I've been pleased with the results because it helps to control my seizures with the most tolerable side effects. I initially experienced some mood swings, became angry, and felt remorse, but they eventually wore off. The other side effect that I have learned to live with is being sleepy, so I try to stay active. The benefits far outweigh the inconvenience of being drowsy. It's important to note this is my personal experience, and yours may be different. So talk to your doctor to find out what's right for you.

In 2002, my doctor talked to me about considering brain surgery—it was rather obvious that I had had an increase in seizure activity as I was getting older. That was no surprise to me because I'd been keeping a detailed journal about my epilepsy—we ended up reviewing it together. However, when my wife was diagnosed with breast cancer, he respected the fact Chris' health was our biggest priority. After my wife's health had improved, we began a series of tests in 2003.

That July, I entered the hospital for a week and this time, within an hour—literally—after I had been hooked up to all the monitoring equipment, I had a seizure—a doozy—caught on tape. In four days, they were able to film at least six very strong seizures. A decision concerning the possibility of surgery was made after multiple MRIs, a PET Scan, neuropsychological exam, and a Wada Test. I was a candidate! And the results of the surgery were positive for me.

As months passed, I was getting more and more excited about the possibility of being able to drive again. Legally, I could have started driving after being seizure free for six months, but the doctors convinced me to wait for a year just to be sure—which I reluctantly agreed to do.

What's Helped Me

• Look at pictures from your past. Write a story about the painful seasons and the joyful seasons of your life. Write a story about what you hope your next life chapter will be. Write a list of ways you can help that chapter become a reality.

Chris Maxwell

Then it happened! Just five days short of a year, the auras started back up. I was really disappointed, yet in a way almost relieved, because I'd been wondering if I could ever trust myself again. Obviously, that's no longer an issue. I threw the driver's license booklet away.

Before the surgery, I averaged dozens of seizures and hundreds of auras a month. Since then, I have experienced mild auras, and only two seizures in which I lost awareness of my surroundings, and only for a few seconds. It's not perfect, but then I don't know anyone whose life is.

So where do I go from here? My parents and Chris and her parents have been my biggest source of human strength. I never would have made it through some of the tough times we faced without their love, help, support, and encouragement. And, on those occasionally rough days, it's encouraging to know that our extended family and close friends have been there all along, doing everything they can to help. Without that help, I don't think I would have made it.

What parts of this story are similar to your story? How do you feel when reading stories about doctors struggling to diagnose cases of epilepsy? What "incident" or "incidents" come to your mind after reading this story? What "help" do you need to "make it?"

14

Surrenders

I woke in bits, like all children, piecemeal over the years. I discovered myself and the world, and forgot them, and discovered them again.[36] —Annie Dillard

We wake, if we ever wake at all, to mysteries, rumors of death, beauty, violence.[37] —Annie Dillard

Every brain has a story and this is mine. . . . By the end of the morning I could not walk, talk, read, write, or recall any of my life. Curled up into a little fetal ball, I felt my spirit surrender to my death, and it certainly never dawned on me that I would ever be capable of sharing my story with anyone.[38] —Jill Bolte Taylor, PhD

Susan Nagy is one of my many friends in this underwater voyage. We are so alike—and so very different. We can understand the struggles we both face, but I cannot understand how she can do so many things well. We meet at epilepsy gatherings and she talks about car engines—she can repair them, and I don't know the names of any parts. She tells me about the meals she cooks for her family—I, uh, will never become a chef. And she works on computers, all while joking about her mental computer's damage. Let her story encourage you.

36 Annie Dillard, *An American Childhood* (New York: HarperCollins, 1987) 10.
37 *Pilgrim at Tinker Creek*, 4.
38 *My Stroke of Insight*, 1.

In September 2002, I was in intensive care for eight days battling meningitis. I came home to a very difficult recovery. I fought daily for three months. Every day was a struggle, even a shower made me tired.

I was first diagnosed with epilepsy in May of 2002, after my friends noticed me zoning out while teaching and talking!

I was determined to keep going after my diagnosis. I continued to work as a technologist in a school, one hour from home, thanks to an amazing group of friends. They drove me back and forth daily. My principal was and still is very understanding. I was blessed.

After a year of various drugs, I worked my way up to 28 pills a day and was told I needed to consider brain surgery. Yikes! Me, a mother of two young boys, brain surgery? I had to have many tests to see if I was a surgical candidate. I needed to have depth electrodes implanted surgically first to make sure they were coming from the right temporal lobe.

Did You Know?

Historically, epilepsy research has been under-funded. Each year NIH spends $30 billion on medical research, but just one half of one percent is spent on epilepsy.

source: cureepilepsy.org/ aboutepilepsy/facts.asp

On November 11, 2004, I had surgery, and, initially, all went smoothly. The bad news was that during surgery, they pierced a vein in my brain and it formed a clot, so they hauled me back into surgery, immediately. When I came out of surgery, I remained hospitalized for fourteen days. I was told I'd have to go back into surgery for the lobectomy *only* when the clot was gone.

This time, I was knocked down, but I went home to recover with my mother, and that's how I learned to be a "patient patient." For two months, I recuperated and waited for the clot to dissipate. *I couldn't even lift a gallon of milk!* But finally, in January 2005, I got the green light for the lobectomy and had the surgery.

My recovery seemed like a long time—about four months, and it included three rounds of steroids to help me recover. And, I have to say, it wasn't exactly pleasant—my brain was so swollen I would hear swooshing. Can you imagine? It was really weird. When they biopsied the four golf ball pieces of my brain they'd removed, they were shocked...I didn't have meningitis. The results showed I had had encephalitis, a potentially life threatening inflammation of the brain. That was a little hard to swallow; finding that I had been misdiagnosed for almost four years.

It was a long recovery. But I have no regrets. After all, brain surgery had its privileges. My brother gave me this beautiful ring the day before I had my lobectomy. He had the word *peace* engraved inside. I had to bust his chops and ask *why*—did you give me this because I'm having a "piece" of my brain removed! Mortified he said, *"No!"* Being the chop buster that I am, I also sent my friends and family an e-mail that had phrases no longer politically correct to say to me, like: Do you have half of a brain? Did you lose your mind? Are you in the right frame of mind (I have no right brain)? I want to give you a piece of my mind . . . and of course, the ever-popular question, Do you have a screw loose?

I still don't think they know if I was kidding or not. On January 10, this year, I was nine years seizure free! I have some memory problems, *but* I have *no* regrets!

Tristin Johnson and I once lived near each other. But we recently became close—though living far apart. That is how it is for many of us with epilepsy. A conversation opens the door for more dialogue. We understand one another. Tristin is a teacher, and I love the thoughts that come through her damaged brain:

From a very early age and before my diagnosis, I can remember the feeling of a partial seizure. I would have a sudden hyper-awareness of time and space, a rising epigastric sensation, an impending sense of doom, and an urge to escape all at the same time.

In an instant, I am separate from the world as we know it. The hustle of everyday lives. The constant pace of morning to night. For a brief moment, my world stands still. I am absorbed with fear and panic but also relieved of everyday rush. I am isolated from all that I know only to awaken and find that I've caught back up with time.

I was diagnosed with Temporal Lobe Epilepsy when I was eight years old, summer of 1993. I received this diagnosis following my first generalized seizure. After that, it was troubleshooting with prescription after prescription. One medication would work for a month or two, but partial and complex partial seizures would always make their return. Secondary generalized seizures were always well under control with any anti-seizure medication but not the partial and complex partial seizures.

During my struggle with epilepsy, I never had someone to relate to. I tried talking to people and sharing my feelings, but no one understood. I poured my heart out to some, but all I got was a blank stare or a comment suggesting I was making it more than it was. Trying to explain epilepsy to someone who doesn't have epilepsy is like speaking a foreign language. I've received countless confused looks.

Throughout my childhood and into adulthood, one question remained on my mind. Why? I questioned why I had to fight a battle with epilepsy. I still find myself asking "why."

Just as I started my final semester of student teaching, I was called to the college professor's office and told to write a letter to all of my students' parents explaining to them that I have epilepsy and assuring them that I was level-headed enough to keep their kids safe. They thought of me as a liability. I was told to do the letter or be dropped from the education program. It was the most humiliating moment of my life. I really could have used a friend who understood my problem.

On November 12, 2008, I had a left temporal lobectomy. That was the beginning of my happily ever after. Since that day, my quality of life has improved tenfold. Everyone has bad days. When I have a bad day, I remind myself that it is not at all as bad as it was before.

I now know what to do with my experience with epilepsy. My struggle with epilepsy was for me to know why it is important for epileptics to form relationships with each other and for me to give to others what I did not have: someone to relate to.

> ## What's Helped Me
>
> · Select ten songs which illustrate various times in your underwater experience. Write about how those songs relate.
>
> **Chris Maxwell**

What parts of their stories remind you of your story? In what ways has your story been hard to swallow? What do the words "long recovery" bring to your mind? How can you take practical steps to help your own underwater story become better? Do you understand the importance of relationships? What are you doing to develop healthy relationships?

15

Songs

In order to come back to the present moment, we must consciously slow down our minds. To do this, first decide you are not in a hurry. Your left mind may be rushing, thinking, deliberating, and analyzing, but your right mind is very m-e-l-l-o-w.[39] —Jill Bolte Taylor, PhD

My right mind understands that I am the life force power of the fifty trillion molecular geniuses crafting my form! (And it bursts into song about that on a regular basis!) It understands that we are all connected to one another in an intricate fabric of the cosmos, and it enthusiastically marches to the best of its own drum.[40] —Jill Bolte Taylor, PhD

I can remember the song lyrics though not recalling the name of the singer. That happens often in this PE (post-encephalitis) life.

On a recent two-hour drive home from the airport, I tested my brain a little. I had just heard stories like those we are reading, and my mind was, again, on my mind. My self-designed exam was to remember the song lyrics—I scored high. On the other portion of the exam—remembering the band or artist singing the song—I scored low. Very low. I'm glad I can't remember how low.

But the ride home and the songs brought back images and stories in my mind. Songs tend to do that. Songs lyrically and musically exhibit images. Songs capture listeners and entice them into a scene.

---

39 *My Stroke of Insight*, 161.
40 Ibid, 141.

The selection of songs took me places as the car took me home. The songs took me to my many other homes—those memories and mysteries and magic, those stories and fun and love, those questions and conflict and solutions.

Like life underwater.

Music becomes reality.

Songs allow listeners to relate though our stories are different from when the lyrics were originally crafted.

Brains recall and imagine. Even a damaged brain can use rhythm and rhyme and tricky phrases to keep nouns and verbs in that place of remembering.

Just like stories. I can relate to stories.

Like Breanne Dancel's story. When she was eight years, old she was in a serious accident in a car being driven by a drunk driver. Left stranded on the side of the road, she was found by a police officer and taken to the closest hospital. Listen to her story like a song as you read her narrative:

> The first hospital I arrived at said I wasn't going to make it or, if I did, I would have been a vegetable. My grandmother and parents didn't believe them, so I was transferred to the best hospital in the United States, Johns Hopkins. In a coma, I was on life support for two months. Thanks to my parents who never stopped believing it was possible for me to survive. From what I was told, my brain was damaged so bad that, at the age of eight, I was a baby all over again. For several months, I had to attend speech and physical therapy, but as time went by, I started to improve. About one year later, I had my first seizure and was diagnosed with epilepsy at the age of nine. Growing up, I was bullied, called a retard, and felt very lonely. I always thought my life was never going to change. Within

What's Helped Me

• Seek to become part of a support group.

• Refuse to make major decisions when you feel emotionally unstable.

• Refuse to let anger control you.

Chris Maxwell

those years, I had so many seemingly impossible challenges that I just wanted to end it all, but because I truly believed in future dreams, I never went down that dark path.

At nineteen, my life changed dramatically when I was introduced to trial medications. I believed anything was worth trying if my doctors believed the future outcome would become better. A few years passed, and I started to feel more freedom with who I was and what I was capable to do. Later, I was introduced to a company that blessed me with friends who also live with epilepsy. With their help, I became more open-minded, and I felt more free to be myself. I never have to hide who I am or keep things a secret because these people are just like me. These friends are the ones who showed me that no matter where you go, life is always worth living. They helped me see it's not about living; it's about what you can give.

Did You Know?

The Federal government spends much less on epilepsy research compared to other diseases, many of which affect fewer people.

source: cureepilepsy.org/ aboutepilepsy/facts.asp

Brain damage, cognitive impairment, memory loss, and epilepsy have taken a toll on my life, *but I never let it hold me back or take me down*. I don't let my epilepsy or disabilities stop me from living a normal life because *I have learned being special is a gift God gives*. These days, I am more open to who I am inside and out. I love telling my story because I love to inspire others to live their lives the way they wish. No matter where you are in this world, remember to stay positive, keep moving forward, know you will always be loved, and you will never be alone.

If you found a song to match her story, what song would you select? What musical style would be a nice fit? She never has to hide anymore. She never keeps a secret anymore.

Now think about your story. How would it sound as a song? How would you sing it? Would your verses include the conflict and tension of life underwater? Would your chorus offer a glimpse of joy? Would the bridge be worth repeating, offering a smile amid the tears?

Or think about Michele Black and her husband, Jesse. I wonder how we could turn her story into a song:

> I began my epilepsy in the fourth grade, and after seven years of seeing doctors, I was finally diagnosed in the eleventh grade. After every anticonvulsant they were able to put me on, four brain operations (which were rare because they included two temporal lobectomies), and several different drug studies, I've been through quite enough to know what I'm talking about.
>
> Epilepsy isn't really all that hard to live with. It's mostly other people that make it so hard to endure. Sometimes, family members, friends, or even total strangers who are uneducated about the disease are what make it so hard to bear. What is most offensive to me is, after all I've been through to get rid of my seizures, someone makes a quite rude comment, stating or implying that I'm only using epilepsy as an excuse to get out of working. When at the same time, I've tried any and all I can to find work. Unfortunately, that's when the uneducated encroach on my life again. So many have stereotyped epilepsy as just one type of seizure alone: falling to the floor, going into convulsions, and trying to swallow your tongue. The type I have are complex partial seizures and not even close to what they expect. They see "epilepsy" on my job application, and even though I had an interview scheduled for the job, my interview is cancelled. I've been told, when they call my interview, "Sorry, but the position has been filled."
>
> I'm about as sick as I can get when I hear the statement, "No, we don't discriminate against people with any medical problems." That's the most bogus comment I've ever heard.

My husband and I have been married thirty-five years. Thankfully, we've been very blessed, and I'm able to get insurance through Jesse's job that accepts "pre-existing" conditions.

Do you hear her tone of voice as you read her story? As she confesses frustration related to the perspective many people have about epilepsy, I don't see her smiling. I detect a rigid look. I hear a frank tone of voice. I spot firm body language.

I would love to do a research study on her story.

I would love to see a good end to where her story goes.

Like the other stories, I would love to hear it as a song. If not literally, I would love to figuratively bring internal music to the scars of our brains, the scars in our relationships, the scars in our hearts.

Music and memory can be friends.

What are your favorite songs? Why do you like them?

What are the songs which best describe your own underwater story? Why did you select those songs?

What part of the song brings tears? What part brings laughter? What part brings hope?

What can you do today, tomorrow, this week, this month, and this year to add a verse of hope to your underwater life song?

Make a list. Select ten goals or steps you can take to pursue a better life now—refusing to be controlled by what you cannot control.

Play the music. Sing the song.

And remember, you are crafting the lyrics yourself.

16

Struggles

It occurred to me that my relationship with statistics changed as soon as I became one.

In her office, I felt like myself, like a self. Outside her office, I no longer knew who I was.[41] —Paul Kalanithi

"How was your doctor appointment?"

"Oh, it was fine. Traffic was bad. I waited a long time before he saw me, but it was fine."

"What did he tell you?"

"Not much, really. He thinks I'm doing okay."

"Did you tell him or the nurse about feeling dizzy again?"

"Yeah."

"What did they say?"

"It's nothing really."

"You don't remember, do you? You don't remember what they said."

"I don't want to talk about this. I don't remember if I said anything about it, okay? I think I did, but I'm not sure. I just don't wanna talk about this."

"I knew I should go with you. Why won't you let me go with you to the doctor? I can help you remember what to say, and I can remember what they say. I'm going with you next time. When is your next appointment? You didn't show me the card."

---

41 *When Breath Becomes Air*, 134, 141.

"I don't want you there. I just want to handle this stuff myself. And I don't remember when my next appointment is."

"Where is the paperwork they gave you?"

"I don't know. Let's talk about it later. I'm going to bed."

No, this is not a fictional conversation. Many readers can relate—they might think it is their dialogue. I'm not including names here, but put yourself there. As the patient. As the caregiver.

The two met with me for counseling after their stress reached a new, and dangerous, level. We went deeper into history, tendencies, mental struggles, emotional wounds, and deep fears. They both carried scars. They both felt, each in their own way, underwater. "No rescue in sight," the caregiver said.

What's Helped Me

· Be aware of the potential dangers of caffeine, alcohol, and various foods.

· If you struggle with an addiction of any type, seek help. Today.

Chris Maxwell

The patient was tired of being told what to do. He felt out of control. That revealed itself in his resistance.

The caregiver was tired of not being allowed to help. She felt the urgency to take over. That revealed itself in her tone of voice and her facial expression.

He looked away.

She stared him in the face.

They were exhausted. They needed help. They needed friends. They needed sleep. They needed a plan.

They needed to be rescued.

What worked for them might not work for you. But please, if you are in a similar battle, seek help. Neurologists and epileptologists aren't always available for every need we face. Their schedules are busy, and their roles are limited. They can, though, refer you to a neuropsychologist. And you can also pursue help with a support group, a counselor, or a minister.

Becky Dennis agrees. She advises:

Find a good therapist in whom you can confide. Be willing to listen. And be willing to be honest with yourself.

The results will work wonders. Did I sound irritable at the beginning of my journey? Yes. But could I recognize it on my own? No. Get a therapist.[42]

Refuse to remain in denial. Do not leave this situation alone—it's not leaving you alone.

For that particular patient and caregiver, they both began a journey of facing their fears. They talked, wrote, confessed, and prayed. They remained silent to hear the other's stories. They voiced to each other honest feelings. While this story doesn't include details from the months of meetings, they finally faced the reality of life underwater—tissues wiped tears, words resurrected wounds, apologies healed hurts, honesty provided air for breath underwater.

The caregiver began to seek a better understanding of feelings instead of limiting her role to only the knowledge of facts and the finding of solutions. The caregiver found new ways to show her care.

The patient finally realized he needed practical assistance in organizing, planning, and remembering. He never went to the doctor alone again. He changed his view. He imagined himself in the place of a caregiver, knowing he might one day become one—for a different reason, in different water, but still there to care for another person.

Their harsh tones began transforming into friendly dialogue. They smiled at each other. Not fake grins to trick observers. Facial expressions where the eyes revealed a gladness to see the other person. Sincere words of admiration. A hug. A nod. Deep tears. Laughter. Appreciation.

They swam together. They faced tension together. They came ashore together.

Underwater for years because of the same storm, they'd drifted into different regions. They needed to meet again and swim ashore.

Together. Helping one another.

They did.

They came ashore together.

---

42 Becky Dennis, *Brain Wreck: A Memoir—A patient's unrelenting journey to save her mind and restore her spirit* (Plano, TX: Majamo Publishing, 2012) 289.

How can you? Do you know the deeper story within the story of your patient or caregiver? What do you fear most? How do you typically or habitually respond to that fear?

The stats and the stories scare me. Too many people like us are giving up too soon. Too many are swimming alone without ever seeking assistance. Too many caregivers have cared so long that they feel there's no need to continue. Too many patients desire to find their value but often choose unhealthy isolation to locate it.

Seek the best help fitting your situation. Refuse to be controlled by the desire to control. Pursue the support group online or in person, the guidance from a medical professional to help you find the help you need, the willingness to no longer stay as you are, the courage to confess a need to change.

Experts can offer great advice. They can guide you. Ask for their help. Today.

Licensed Clinical Psychologist Blake Rackley, PsyD, offers practical advice for caregivers:

1. You are not alone as a caregiver. While your child, spouse, parent, or friend is the patient, you have to know your limits as well. Many organizations provide respites for those caregivers who simply need a break. There are camps for those children who have seizures that are often free, which gives a caregiver a chance to recuperate.

2. Seek counseling. During the years that I have counseled children who have epilepsy, I have noticed that many of the parents are tired, anxious, and/or depressed. They wanted more for their child. They are worried about the future of their child and even their own future. They are worried about what it means for their child to live a normal life, and this, in turn, elicits some depression. As your child goes to different therapies, doctors, and neurologists, you may need some help as well. You do not have to be strong all the time.

3. It is okay for you to feel weak. As I have talked with spouses and adult children of those who have epilepsy, I have noticed the reoccurring theme that they feel that they have to always be strong. Create a support system around you who understands your struggle. Have a break during the week where you are with friends and family.

4. Know that you can't control everything or find an explanation for everything that happens. Epilepsy is an unpredictable disorder,

which makes us feel scared and often alone. You work and work and seemingly get everything under control, and then one seizure sets you back to square one. It will leave you feeling frustrated and defeated. This is where a good psychologist, counselor, and/or pastor can help you. Support groups can allow you to vent and feel connected.

5. Do not allow the disorder to disrupt your day to day life and your ability to have fun. Many people feel afraid to go out and live because they may have a seizure. While proper precautions can be made (cell phone, medical bracelets, information on what to do in your pocket or purse), do not live in fear. Remember that, while this disorder is unpredictable at times, you must live life and find happiness.

6. Do not allow the disorder to rule everything you do, especially spending time together working on your marriage. Many parents center their lives around caring for their child and forget to care about each other, which creates strangers in their own homes. While the disorder is life changing/altering, it is not always life "ending." Please know that I say the last part with sensitivity and an understanding that many have had their lives taken by the disorder. I'm simply saying that there is a difference between living life and simply surviving day after day.

> ### What's Helped Me
> • Go on a retreat. Rest. Reflect on your life. Realize your importance. Release hurts in healthy ways. Rethink your condition. Realign your priorities. Renew your commitments and guidelines. Rejoice and be glad. Reenter your normal routine with inner healing, fresh vision, and new energy.
>
> *Chris Maxwell*

Sherri Carey has been a wonderful help for me at my job. Like those who worked for me years ago, she has found ways to adjust to my unadjustable self.

She says it has also helped her to work with me because of her husband's story. I can help her, the caregiver, understand from a patient's perspective.

Sherri tells us a little bit about her situation:

He had a major heart attack with a 100 percent blockage, and his heart went into v-fib. He suffered oxygen loss which caused brain damage. The damage includes short-term memory loss and involuntary movements. This happened in the early hours of December 17, 2009. He was a normal fifty-two-year-old man who was highly intelligent with an awesome witty sense of humor. Very detailed- and work-oriented with many musical talents, he sang all the time and played his guitar. You could set your watch by him and his daily habits. He loved to joke and pick on people.

Everyone loves him because he is so easy to love. He got along with everyone. He is still loved by everyone. But now he no longer sings. He hardly ever jokes. He is completely opposite. Nothing drives him. He has no ability for detail, and he cannot remember certain things—like if he fed the dogs or if he asked you a question. He is still very loving and caring. In fact, he is more openly loving and caring now.

Our whole world was and has been turned upside down. Our income was drastically changed. Now we have to watch what we spend. I am now the only one who pays bills or really does anything. This is very stressful for me. I have no one now to help make decisions with. Even though I am not alone, it feels like I am at times. Through this whole journey, when I could not find the answer or couldn't figure it out, God always showed up. He has been with me step by step and has showed Himself to me in many different ways. He has always had an answer for me.

My advice for others is to not give up. When I felt all alone and that there was no hope, it always showed up. You just have to keep your eyes and mind open to what God has in store for you!

What's Helped Me

- Give time or money or encouraging words to a business or agency helping people with special needs.

Chris Maxwell

17

Side Effects

I don't want to still be mad ten years from now. I don't want to be unable to talk about it, or have it all come out of me in another way, like suddenly I don't like children anymore because I lost one, and I could never face it.[43] —Christopher de Vinck

"I read the signs aright," he said to himself. "Frodo ran to the hill-top. I wonder what he saw there? But he returned by the same way, and went down the hill again."[44] — J.R.R. Tolkien

"You can't take it with you," the old statement claims.

But we often can. And we do.

We take with us what we choose to carry. Unnecessary luggage of past pain often travels with us in our sail. We hold tightly to that statement about our failure, our appearance, our inability, our disability.

We also take with us side effects of various anti-epileptic drugs, or treatments received to help defeat or endure other health issues. We carry with us scar tissue and forgetfulness. We carry with us weights we fail to remember we are carrying.

Anna Kitchens wrote a story for me about her own luggage. I battle a war in the brain—feeling off in the sea alone. She battles a war in the brain a different

---

43 Christopher de Vinck, *The Power of the Powerless: A Brother's Legacy of Love* (New York: Doubleday, 1988) 65.
44 J.R.R. Tolkien, *The Lord of the Rings, Part Two: The Two Towers* (New York: Ballantine Books, 1965) 17.

way—feeling unworthy and unimportant and unbeautiful. As you read her story, think about the side effects of how you've learned from, or refused to learn from, your own battles.

I finally was at a place where I knew it would be detrimental to my health if I didn't seek help and healing. So with the nudging of my closest two friends, I told my counselor what was going on, and from there, we started recovery. I wish I could say that that's when it started getting better, but it's not that simple. I would still go from restricting food, to purging, to sleeping all of the time in hopes of avoiding the issue all together. For the entire last half of the semester, I had one of my closest friends either be with me while I ate, or I would be required to send her snapchats of my meals, so that she could sign off on my food log for counseling. I felt like a five-year-old and was so frustrated and angry that out of everything I could be dealing with so badly, it was food.

> **What's Helped Me**
>
> · Become friends with someone who has an illness similar to yours. Encourage each other.
>
> *Chris Maxwell*

Also, in the midst of all of this, I was preparing to go on my first mission trip—to Tanzania, Africa.

I went to Tanzania in June, and for two weeks, my life changed. I was with people who didn't know me and was in a completely different place. I felt like while I was there, I had permission to be normal. I could eat normally, and no one would suspect anything because no one knew of my struggle. The last day in Tanzania, after an amazing two weeks, I began to have a lot of fear and anxiety about going back home because I thought it would all be the same as before I left. But I heard God say to me, *"Am I not the same God at home as I am here in Tanzania? I transcend all of the boundaries."*

I came back home, and the rest of my summer was an emotional and spiritual "high." I started the first semester of my senior year in August, and until a few weeks ago, I had never had a better semester. But a couple of weeks ago, that started to shift. Food has become a huge point of anxiety again, and to be honest, I was super disappointed. I genuinely thought that it was over for good, and that I had been healed. But even still, I feel like there is this ongoing conversation between me and God, and it has gone something like this:

Me: God, why? Is this really going to be forever? Am I never going to be completely healed? Is this a permanent mental illness I will have forever? There's medicine for depression and anxiety. . . . There's no medicine for this. Why this? Why is this so hard for me? Please help. I just want to be okay again...

GOD: I am still God. I am still good. I am still faithful. I am strong enough, when you're not. Even if it doesn't completely go away the way you think it should, know that this is not who you are. You are Mine. You are healed. Seasons change, but even so—I do not.

I think that's where I am at in my story right now. I know God is able to heal me and make this issue not an issue in my life anymore, but even if He doesn't, He will be with me, and I won't be broken because of this. Eventually, I will be okay.

Are you "finally at a place?" Are you ready to start recovery—of denial, of addiction, of emotional and mental side effects of life with epilepsy, of years of fear from a life underwater?

Anna said, "I felt like while I was there, I had permission to be normal." Today, I want to realize that my normal is my normal, and it is an okay normal, a good normal, a normal with a future. Today, I want you to realize your normal is your normal, and it is an okay normal, a good normal, a normal with a future.

No, this is not a method of defending damaging tendencies. It is not giving an excuse for refusing to seek help. It is the view luring us *toward* help. Amid the inner wars, we can be us. We can seek help. We can pray prayers. We can visit people underwater in another country. We can serve the hurting and refuse to live obsessed with our own battles. We can, through life, fight for another person instead of letting our own battles own us.

Anna found hope through facing her situation, seeking counsel, accepting accountability, visiting a doctor, and praying to her God.

How can you find hope today?

Hope is not hiding far away as you might think. It is close. It is near. It is available.

A website, a support group, a doctor, a counselor, a life coach, a friend, a mentor, a walk in the rain. A song, a book, a walk on the beach. Writing a journal, making a call, staring at the mirror and smiling back. A deep breath, a slow walk, a swim in the ocean of reality and choosing to embrace your situation. During sensory overload, uncontrolled seizures, unanswered questions, forgotten names, and frustrating medical results, pursue hope by seeking help. Refuse to swim alone.

Though not always simple, we can find ways that work for each of us.

I've always preferred routine. That tendency reached a new level of success, as I like to label it, after my illness.

Before encephalitis, I was a picky eater who always arrived early, paid bills early, and failed to understand why others weren't early. After the illness, those virtues, another selfish word choice, reached new levels of success. Life is crafted into time slots. Food dwells in me as a limited tribe of selections. On time is spelled "early." And interruptions disrupt my crafted concentration and conversation.

That's me. My story, my struggle, my disability.

What is yours?

One friend tells me how she sees herself when she looks in the mirror. She doesn't like what she says. Years of skipping food or vomiting are catching up. She feels underwater.

The doctor said the word a friend dreaded: cancer. His life has never been the same. He feels underwater.

The spouse said goodbye. You knew things weren't the same, and you wondered what else was happening. But you didn't expect this. Not now, anyway. How will you tell the children? What will it do to them? To you?

The boss called you into his office and told you the news. What job will you pursue now?

The alcohol wouldn't leave your mind. You'd gone thirty-seven days without a drink. But the desire was too strong that night. You drank. And drank more. Then drove home. All your friends watched the story in the news. What now?

The images look and feel real. No rejection. Just the picture and the thrill. You never believed you'd become addicted to porn for a decade.

The job is fun. It covers your schedule, but you feel like a success. They love you there. They reward you there. But do your children even know you?

Every other couple can have kids. Why can't you?

Every other friend finds a spouse. Why can't you?

Every other student seems to make good grades and complete assignments well. Why can't you?

Every other friend can sleep without a pill. Why can't you?

Every other friend can stop eating before overeating. Why can't you?

> **What's Helped Me**
> · Become friends with someone who has a struggle very different from yours. Learn from one another.
> *Chris Maxwell*

Every other friend can stay in a relationship without finding a reason to escape before feelings become too intense and commitment becomes too serious. Why can't you?

You're afraid of heights. Or elevators. Or small rooms. Or honest conversations. Or deep relationships. Or the future. Or seeing a counselor. Or eating a meal. Or stopping work to take a nap. Or waking up to face a new day.

Feeling underwater, feeling trapped in that region below the surface, scares you.

But remember: Much occurs underwater. We can map oceans' floors. We can learn of them through our technology. We can visit but not stay. Survival underwater is limited because of the lack of oxygen.

For the moment, think of your own underwater survival. Absorbing the sunlight. Feeling the freezing temperature. Seeking oxygen. Sharks, dolphins, crabs, seashells, salmon, and pet fish. The underwater habitat hasn't always been pleasant.

They assured you the financial decision would succeed. It didn't. Now, you know this word so well: debt.

You prayed. And prayed. And prayed. Your friends assured you healing would come. It didn't. Words at the funeral about "now healed forever" do not take away the pain. Now you know this word: death.

The sinkhole. The hurricane. The fires. The lightning every afternoon.

Reactionary? Desensitized? Enabling?

I listened to Elaine Dowell, MBE Founder of the Encephalitis Society UK, talking about me. About us. She explained synapses—electrical impulses via transmitter molecules. She emphasized about the importance of calming down. She taught me how to "keep the cars off the network if they aren't needed or they'll block the road." She provided information about molecules, how memory finds a match, synchronicity, circuits, embedded, forming of memory, frequency embedded network into brain, how a wall normally protects the brain to keep it so well protected, how viruses are small and can get into the nerve cells easier than bacteria, how it is like a terrorist attack, how before rebuilding things need to be cleaned out, how to start rebuilding. She used words and phrases like face recognition, neurons, network, retract, regenerating, frail, some nerves will fail, big gap, parts will be broken, lost connections when tired and during times of stress, post-synaptic neuron, when molecules aren't working, how trying to work through it isn't good, how to stop before you get tired, that when you're tired, it is too late, how to listen to your brain, how caregivers can notice.

I talked to her after the session. She said, "A brain is shutting down because it wants to rest. Your brain has been injured. That is part of what you are now—moving forward with the disease is coming to terms with who you are now."

But how? "Rest again. Stop doing so much. Setbacks are common—you can no longer do what you formerly could do. Eat fresh fruit, exercise, be sure your activity is followed by rest—close your eyes and rest, do meditation. Accept that you are fragile."

I read the stories by Debbie Hampton on her Web site, The Best Brain Possible. Her advice and encouragement help me swim in my mental war at sea. They can help us all—whatever our cause for life underwater.

18

Schedules

When you finally see what goes on underwater, you realize that you've been missing the whole point of the ocean. Staying on the surface all the time is like going to the circus and staring at the outside of the tent.[45] —Dave Barry

One of the things I know about writing is this: spend it all, shoot it, play it, lose it, all, right away, every time. Do not hoard what seems good for a later place in the book or for another book; give it, give it all, give it now. The impulse to save something good for a better place later is the signal to spend it now. Something more will arise for later, something better. These things fill from behind, from beneath, like well water. Similarly, the impulse to keep to yourself what you have learned is not only shameful, it is destructive. Anything you do not give freely and abundantly becomes lost to you. You open your safe and find ashes.[46] —Annie Dillard

I despise being interrupted. When speaking my portion of a conversation, an interruption, though well-intended, becomes a thief breaking in and robbing my mind.

When interrupted, I feel lost at sea. My location isn't it easy to find. Where was that? Where am I? How do I locate myself again, and my word again, and my thoughts again?

---

45 Dave Barry, "Blub story a very deep experience," Miami Herald February 19, 1989.
46 Annie Dillard, *The Writing Life* (New York: HarperCollins, 1989) 78.

An interruption becomes the conclusion. My verbal adventure stops suddenly. A wall appears. Another step feels impossible. I wait and wait and wait for an opening, for a memory, for a word. Nothing emerges.

Finally, I locate another word as a substitute.

Or I ask for help.

Either way, I do not like this.

But I'm learning this.

I am learning this life—this life of failure, of frustrations, of dependence, of forgetting. This life of interruptions. This life with baggage. This life at sea. I'm adjusting to this life of always knowing a seizure is possible. This life with epilepsy.

It feels like a caution light blinking and blinking. Do I stop or slow? Do I turn?

I choose, usually, to not frown when facing those facts. I smile. People with epilepsy have boundaries, but don't all people? Yes, we need sleep and the care of others and sunglasses, but all people do. We need the caution light's reminder of these words: be careful. All people do. We are unique yet not controlled by our conditions.

Well, let's get back to the interruptions. Words, often difficult to locate in this brain, frequently take time to be stated. Much time. I try. They hide. I try hard. They refuse to reveal themselves. A noun. A name of a person I know. A verb. An action I've known well and long. Hidden, distant, afar: words.

I merge memories and mingle experiences. I try. I fail to find words.

But the process is worse when interrupted. Let me try and fail, then ask for a name. Don't invade my endeavor to recall.

Though, if I sat in your seat and listened to my weak attempt to remember, if I stared at a frustrated face like my own and craved to offer assistance, I would interrupt. I'd bid a solution if the situation was opposite. I get it.

But I'm helped best when those close to me realize they'll never fully get it. They just choose to endure the wait—hearing my conversation stop, seeing

---

What's Helped Me

• Find artwork which encourages you. Look at it often.

Chris Maxwell

---

my facial expressions of frustration, desiring to rescue me from the war of forgetfulness, hurting with me—while hidden words merge their appearance slowly if at all.

Give me a little time even if I request otherwise.

Give me a little time even when my search engine malfunctions.

Give me a little time until I can invest no more effort in the adventure of recall.

Give me time underwater.

And, please, give me your acceptance even when my attempts to remember or stay calm or seem normal all fail.

When rough waters and fierce storms interrupt our lives, our schedules will never be the same. The ruthless waves invaded our ordinary life novel.

So I think of the one in twenty-six people in the United States who have epilepsy at some time in their lives. I think of their interruptions—their seizures, their moods, their emotions. I think of their schedules, now including doctor appointments and tests and naps.

I also think of you. I wonder: who is reading this, and what is his or her story? What is your storm? What interrupted your calm swim near the shore? What has taken you deep into frightening portions of unfamiliar territory?

I think of Vernon Anderson's story of his wife dying and his adventure of raising a son with special needs. I think of Bryan Griffin choosing to ride his bike long distances as therapy and exercise in his epilepsy adventure. I think of Tim and Marie Kuck's five years of Nathaniel's life with various special needs.

And I think of you. Who is there to help you? Are you allowing their help?

And I think of the many people I need to thank. Ray for mowing the grass and taking over our yards while I recovered. Garrett for being there when I needed someone. My accountability guys for helping me adjust to a partly cloudy life. A church for loving the first me and the second me. My wife and her family. Our sons. My two sisters and my dad—and memories of our mom who died when my nineteen-year-old brain didn't warn us that I needed her to stay around for my ocean encounter. Those who drove me when I couldn't drive even though it—or, I—drove them crazy. The office workers and staff and board members who brought stability during the rapid currents.

Patti, my speech therapist, I thank you. The students who learned how to do speech therapy by working with this underwater guy—after our insurance incorrectly assumed I needed no more help. They were wrong. But you were there. Thank you. "Speech therapy is an art that deserves to be more widely known. You cannot imagine the acrobats your tongue mechanically performs in order to produce all the sounds of a language."[47]

My doctors and nurses. My counselors. My students. My editors and publishers and marketing teams. Thank you.

Those who endured me in Florida. Those who welcomed me in Georgia. Those who've invited me to tell my story. Those who've asked me to listen to their stories. Thank you.

Those who can relate to my story and those who can't. Those who hope to become part of a new season of offering hope to others who have epilepsy. Thank you.

Thank you. Thank you. Thank you.

Those busy in the medical field who still know the importance of seven seconds of eye contact—even though you are demanded to stare at the screen and complete the data, a brief face-to-face chat is like medicine to us. Thank you for looking at us.

Those pharmaceutical companies who have invested in antiepileptic medications to aggressively pursue help. Thank you for seeking a seizure-free life for the future of people with epilepsy.

Giving thanks fits actually. I'm writing this very early in the morning on a day known as Thanksgiving. So what else should I ask that we do, but give thanks?

Though our underwater stories aren't always smiley, perfect, hand-holding journeys of rejoicing, let's take a moment and find things we're thankful for.

Join me and give thanks. For friends and family, give thanks. For doctors and nurses and caregivers, give thanks. For medications and research and better days in the future, give thanks. For water to drink and stars to notice and songs to hear and pictures to see, give thanks. For forgiveness and laughter and long walks and short jogs, give thanks. For modern technology and global contact, give thanks. For research being done and creative minds at work, give thanks. For a better future for those suffering from various illnesses, give thanks. For this moment, right now, give thanks.

---

47   Jean-Dominique Bauby, *The Diving Bell and the Butterfly* (Vintage International, 1997) 40.

Thankful hearts can help our brains. Dwelling on the negatives isn't the best medication to take. Being grateful of small things helps us shift our focus and see life from a better perspective.

Giving thanks isn't denial. Though underwater, we've worked to notice reality. There is too much silence in our world about encephalitis and epilepsy and traumatic brain injury and SUDEP.[48] We are raising our voices and informing the world. We are telling our stories and inviting others to tell theirs.

But as we speak, and as we cry, as we reveal scary information and remember stormy nights, we can add a little gratefulness to the dialogue. Our faces can include a few smiles. Our stories can add a few sentences of thankfulness.

On this Thanksgiving, I looked back at pictures from my first Thanksgiving after encephalitis. I thank our friends for inviting us to New York.

I remember Thanksgivings with my mom's family and my dad's family, with my family. Sad Thanksgivings and joyful Thanksgivings, I recall the meals and football games and snow. I remember forgetting and still being loved.

And I am thankful!

Today, and every day, say "thank you" to someone. Smile at them. Speak with kindness from a deep region of your inner self.

What's Helped Me

• Grab the channel selector and turn off the TV. Stand up. Go outside (or to a different room inside if the weather is bad) and notice reality. Remind yourself about the beauty and wonder and hope. See the stars. Feel the wind. Listen to the traffic. Smile at the puppy walking by. Notice the rabbit or the train track or the deer or the airplane flying over or the bird flying from her nest or the old house or the new house. Refuse to stare at a screen so much that you miss the splendor nearby.

Chris Maxwell

---

48 SUDEP is the sudden, unexpected death of someone with epilepsy, who was otherwise healthy. In SUDEP cases, no other cause of death is found when an autopsy is done. Each year, more than one out of one thousand people with epilepsy die from SUDEP.

And live with a thankful heart.

While you swim through rough waves in this underwater season, tell yourself there is beauty nearby. Notice it, and be thankful for it.

So interrupt today by giving thanks. That interruption might help us all recall our value.

19

Suggestions

As the years passed, I began to learn more and more about the subtleties of compassion and guidance.[49] —Christopher de Vinck

Remember the four words: you are not alone.[50] —Bob Beaudine

Interesting timing. I visited the dentist this morning while I'm writing a book about life with epilepsy. And dentist offices are not always the most enjoyable encounters for people—especially those of us prone to have seizures.

The lighting, the stress, the closed atmosphere, the be-still-and-don't-dare-move facial expressions were never friendly to me after my illness. Before that, I was okay having my teeth worked on. But post-encephalitis, my visits to the dentist included these odd encounters—what I later learned were certain types of seizures.

I'm much more aware now of my triggers. I'm also grateful to be in a better environment—the small town feeling where the workers speak to you and show true care. I stay calm, listening to the music. If I feel something strange, I choose to change where I keep my mental focus. I know the potential danger of certain lights, and I always have my sunglasses with me. The workers know to only use the bright lights when necessary. They've shown me so much kindness—unlike how my concerns were ignored in another office.

---

49 *The Power of the Powerless*, 145.
50 Bob Beaudine, *2 Chairs: The Secret That Changes Everything* (Franklin, TN: Worthy, 2016) 58.

How can others learn from them? One thing they've done is to learn from patients like me. They've asked for advice. They've noticed my tendencies, my fears, my struggles. They've chosen to not hurry.

They make eye contact. They ask questions and actually listen to our answers.

I discussed with them the potential danger of lighting, of stressful places, of tension and seizures, of brain damage and memory, of me—the guy who wasn't stressed visiting dentists pre-illness. I've told them my stories as they opened my mouth to clean and check and send me on my way.

What's Helped Me

• Use your non-dominant hand to brush your teeth, reach for your keys, tie your shoes, write, draw, use the remote and other common actions. This can strengthen neural connections, and possibly grow new ones.

Chris Maxwell

What if more places were that friendly? What if all businesses learned how to make those of us with epilepsy more comfortable and safe? What if we all worked together to learn about other illnesses, disabilities, needs, dangers, and feelings about life underwater?

One area that has always helped me smile is friends. True friends. Friends who accepted the old me and the new me. Friends who welcome the me with epilepsy and a damaged brain.

Friends—fortunately I had, and have, many. Before I almost died, life for me and my family included friends. Meals together. Time in each other's homes, at each other's jobs. Learning together, laughing together, playing sports together, enjoying music together, grieving together.

During the illness and recovery, the after me becoming a much different me, I still had friends. They cared. They showed their care.

I felt alone underwater. But though I felt that way, and though my friends could never fully relate, they cared. They refused to leave me alone.

But many patients are alone.

I want to see that change.

If you are a patient or a caregiver, pursue a support group. If you are not familiar with epilepsy or any type of traumatic brain injury, learn about it. Find people who need a smile. Visit them. Show that you care.

Those are a few suggestions about your visit to the dentist and a few thoughts about people needing people. Because I'm in that mood, here are more of what has helped me.

Just remember, I am not a doctor. *Underwater* isn't a medical journal. My confessions are not advice from an expert. But this story has taught me many lessons. Here are some suggestions that have helped me:

- Rest well and often.

- Drink water.

- Exercise. If walking is all you can do, walk gladly.

- Do not procrastinate.

- Write to remember, to release emotions, to think, to remind someone you care for them.

- Look in the mirror, and believe the person looking back is important.

- Forgive those who have hurt you. Refuse to let pains from the past control your present and future decisions.

- Do not assume forgiving means approving of improper behavior. Do not accept harm (physically or verbally) from someone else. Get away from them. But do not let bitterness travel with you.

- Find the right person to talk to: counselor, life coach, mentor, pastor, friend.

- Schedule times of relaxation—don't wait to see if they show up.

- Dream big.

- Be faithful in everyday tasks, and find pleasure during the routine.

- If you need to (even if it hurts your ego—I said if you "need to," not if you "want to"), let a family member or trusted friend go with you to the doctor. They can help you remember what to tell the doctor and help you remember what the doctor tells you.

- Use modern devices to evaluate and maintain your diet, exercise, budget, time management, medications, and schedules.

- Listen to the sound of silence.

- Breathe deeply and slowly.

- Notice the wonder nearby.

- Keep a list of your medical history and present condition, medications you are taking and medications to avoid, times and dosages of those medications you are taking, names and numbers of people to contact (family, doctors, neighbors, friends, etc.) when needed, and other vital information.

- Read. If reading is difficult because of brain damage, listen to the audio version of books and talks. Keep the mind thinking.

- Find other ways to exercise the brain. Seek to remember and repeat. Take tests. Listen to statements you hear on TV or radio or online and try to repeat each word. Try to memorize portions of songs, books, poems, quotes, and stories. And remember: refuse to get down on yourself when you don't do well. This is working and helping the brain, not testing or condemning the brain.

- Keep sunglasses nearby if you are sensitive to lighting.

- Watch the sun rise.

- Watch the sun set.

- Begin each day with a time of reflection. Set a few goals.

- Hit pause in the middle of each day. Breathe deeply. Reflect and realize: even through the pain and difficulties, you are here and you are important.

- End each day with a time of reflection. Evaluate your efforts to accomplish the goals. If you failed, forgive yourself, and plan ways to achieve those goals in the future.

- Notice your biggest fears. Seek help in learning from those fears and overcoming them.

- Notice your deepest worries. Learn what causes those worries but refuse to be controlled by them.

- Allow yourself to cry.

- Allow yourself to laugh.

- Allow yourself to schedule times to rest the brain and the body.

- Be quick to hear.[51]

- Be slow to talk.

- Be slow to become angry.

- Do not go to sleep angry. Find healthy ways (journaling, praying, seeing a counselor, etc.) of refusing to hold the anger inside or using it to attack someone.[52]

- Look at pictures from your past. Write a story about the painful seasons and the joyful seasons of your life. Write a story about what you hope your next life chapter will be. Write a list of ways you can help that chapter become a reality.

- Select ten songs which illustrate various times in your underwater experience. Write about how those songs relate.

- Seek to become part of a support group.

- Refuse to make major decisions when you feel emotionally unstable.

- Refuse to let anger control you.

> **What's Helped Me**
>
> • Close your eyes and imagine visiting the beauty underwater. Visualization can let your brain take you places. Swim there. Smile there. Be there.
>
> *Chris Maxwell*

- Be aware of the potential dangers of caffeine, alcohol, and various foods.

- If you struggle with an addiction of any type, seek help. Today.

- Go on a retreat. Rest. Reflect on your life. Realize your importance. Release hurts in healthy ways. Rethink your condition. Realign your priorities. Renew your commitments and guidelines. Rejoice and be glad. Reenter your normal routine with inner healing, fresh vision, and new energy.

---

51 Chris will often use the Bible verse, James 1:19—Wherefore, my beloved brethren, let every man be swift to hear, slow to speak, slow to wrath (KJV)— to help him focus on these areas.

52 Chris has found the Bible verse, Ephesians 4:26— Be ye angry, and sin not: let not the sun go down upon your wrath (KJV)—to be good advice in any and all relationships.

- Give time or money or encouraging words to a business or agency helping people with special needs.

- Become friends with someone who has an illness similar to yours. Encourage each other.

- Become friends with someone who has a struggle very different from yours. Learn from one another.

- Find artwork which encourages you. Look at it often.

- Grab the channel selector and turn off the TV. Stand up. Go outside (or to a different room inside if the weather is bad) and notice reality. Remind yourself about the beauty and wonder and hope. See the stars. Feel the wind. Listen to the traffic. Smile at the puppy walking by. Notice the rabbit or the train track or the deer or the airplane flying over or the bird flying from her nest or the old house or the new house. Refuse to stare at a screen so much that you miss the splendor nearby.

- Use your non-dominant hand to brush your teeth, reach for your keys, tie your shoes, write, draw, use the remote and other common actions. This can strengthen neural connections, and possibly grow new ones.

What's Helped Me

- Repeat statements you hear.
- Exercise the brain by playing crossword puzzles and other game.

Chris Maxwell

- Close your eyes and imagine visiting the beauty underwater. Visualization can let your brain take you places. Swim there. Smile there. Be there.

- Repeat statements you hear.

- Exercise the brain by playing crossword puzzles and other games.

- Remember this word: NEW. Select a new hobby. Try to learn a new language. Listen to a new song. Work to learn a new skill.

- Remember this word: OLD. Write what you remember from an old movie or an old song or an old city. Revisit a place of your past and work to recall your season underwater there.

- Play a sport. For fun and growth, not stressful competition. And remember your limitations.

- Drive—or if you aren't able to drive, ask your driver to drive—a different route home. Refuse to always take the same roads at the same time. (This one is very hard for me. Not only because am I a man of habit, but it also helps me not forget. Still, I have learned a few new turns bring me a fresh look and also help my brain. Give it a try.)

This collection of ideas is important for patients. All patients.

And for caregivers. All caregivers.

And for those in the medical field who are so busy caring for the rest of us that they often forget the importance of rest for themselves.

Read through it again. How does it fit your life? What have you neglected? When can you begin a few small steps toward a better future? What might keep you from doing that? Add to the list. Write your own list. Whatever your age and whatever your story, find helpful actions to direct you toward better health and protect you from poor decisions.

See the ideas as priorities. Self-care isn't selfishness. It helps us adjust to our present weakness and reach our greatest potential. It helps us no longer be controlled by what we can't control.

Give your list a name. An inspiring name. A name you can remember. A name which will motivate you to take regular steps toward wholeness. A name which gives you a smile, a nod, a drive. A name to help you no longer live *Underwater*.

20

Spoons

Although it may seem that a lot is known about the origin and treatment of epilepsy, much more is still to be learned.[53]
—Carl W. Bazil, MD, PhD

You also need to take responsibility for your care.[54] —Carl W. Bazil, M.D. PhD

I held the spoon in my hand. Instead of hurrying to fill it with food, I just held it.

My mind again hit reverse. Thoughts went back to my encounter two decades ago and many miles away. I don't remember the event, but I've heard Debbie tell me many times about having to teach me to eat again.

But Debbie wasn't with me this time. I was alone, holding a spoon.

I stared at the silver circle's shining reflection from the straight line. I wasn't confused this time about how to eat—now I am a more obsessive compulsive, keep-my-hands-clean guy than someone who might eat spaghetti or ice cream by hand. These days I still love the ice cream. And eat it with a spoon.

I liked the spoon.

It reminded me of how the word *spoons* was redefined by Christine Miserandino in her essay "The Spoon Theory."[55]

It reminded me how we all need to be careful what, and how much, we carry. We should keep our spoons of life small. Too big and we've packed our voyage

---

53 *Living Well With Epilepsy*, 173.
54 Ibid, 223.
55 https://butyoudontlooksick.com/category/the-spoon-theory/

with unneeded luggage. Things like blame and condemnation and self-hate and self-harm and defiance and performance and gossip and abandonment and rejection and ranking: our life spoons are too tiny to carry those items. Things like skipping medication doses or refusing to bring a helpful caregiver to the doctor with us or refusing to ask more questions to obtain better information or denying the reality of our condition: our life spoons are too tiny to carry those objects. Things like doing everything for everybody all the time: our life spoons are too tiny to carry those things.

If something is too much to carry, let's ask for help. Or simply leave it behind.

I'm not promoting selfishness. I'm suggesting wisdom.

I'm not saluting rebellion. I'm recommending boundaries.

I like to be liked. But I have realized I will not always fit in this world of do-everything-all-day-at-all-times-and-for-everyone-everywhere-every-moment.

Saying no allows me to keep my spoon light.

It also allows me space to say yes at what is best for my health and what I am best at.

> **What's Helped Me**
>
> · Remember this word: NEW. Select a new hobby. Try to learn a new language. Listen to a new song. Work to learn a new skill.
>
> *Chris Maxwell*

This isn't suggesting we hatefully demand our own way. We shouldn't use a harsh tone of voice and excuse ourselves for selfish gains.

But we can gently and calmly say no. We can explain why, without taking it too personally if the other person or people don't understand our spoon.

We probably wouldn't understand theirs either.

I remember Brittany, my daughter-in-law, starting a word game with the family. I can't recall which game, and I can't recall our location. But I remember my initial resistance—two key words that aren't a game; two key words to my recovery and survival. Initial resistance.

Fear can trigger initial resistance. Bad experiences from the past. Doubt. Self-talk. Responses from other people. Many factors can cause initial resistance.

For me, I did not want to play a game where words must be located in a brief amount of time, where competition is included, where memory is crucial, where others observe your mental conflict.

Competition never bothered me before. In sports, in debate, in stating a case. Nor with words. I knew them, I found them, I said them, I wrote them. But that's not how things work post illness. I now know the war of finding words.

I recently discussed that event with Brittany. She thought I would love the game because of my talent with words. Debbie reminded me those experiences are good to help work the brain. They're both correct. But I do better alone when no one gazes at my mental search. Or on stage when telling stories from deep in my heart. Or on mornings like this—awake before anyone else, typing at a pace matching the mental motion, swimming in a sea of my rhythm.

No one grading now. No one reading yet. Just me. A morning. And words.

But sometimes, I need to play the game. Sometimes, we all need to face our fears and frustrations. Sometimes, we need to stand before the crowd and forget. Then laugh. Then love. Then accept the new us, whether those around us do or not.

Failing in a game might be succeeding. Losing might be winning. Forgetting might be remembering that the perfection should not control us.

What's Helped Me

• Remember this word: OLD. Write what you remember from an old movie or an old song or an old city. Revisit a place of your past and work to recall your season underwater there.

Chris Maxwell

Remember, our brains are encountering road work. Our thoughts exit their normal roads, taking different routes. It takes longer to arrive at the destination of a word, a thought, a name. The construction will never conclude.

But we choose to accept life that way. And to be okay with ourselves.

How?

Talk to a counselor or peer about areas of initial resistance. Make a list of your fears. Stare at the words. Dare yourself to face them. Refuse to deny them, but also refuse to be controlled by them.

Pursue victory in a larger game. Choose to swim through your initial resistance. Locate beauty underwater. Replace initial resistance with internal resolve: swim.

With the help of so many others, I learned to swim in this life underwater. I'm still learning how to say yes and how to say no, how to accept myself and refuse to live in comparison, how to find beauty even underwater.

I thought again about hopefulness among hurt when I listened to our son Aaron and his wife tell their stories of caring for children in a foreign land. His compassion and courage merged. Would he be coaching those young men in a difficult land if he had never traveled in this underwater adventure? I don't know. But I do know this. He, and those who have been there for him, have chosen the right spoons. They have left the unneeded luggage behind.

You can too. Through the storms of encephalitis and epilepsy, or your own brain damage or heart damage or relational damage or health damage or disability, you can. Through the automobile accidents and the cancer reports, the fires and wars, the domestic violence and aging, the forgetfulness and remembering what you wish you could forget, you can. Through grief for the dying and grief for the living who have changed so much, you can.

I know that I have "issues." I have weaknesses and battles. I make mistakes. I have brain damage and live with epilepsy. I take medication and forget names. I am a picky eater, and being on time, for me, means arriving very early. I care too much and try too hard. I pull for the Braves.

Those are just a few of my issues, but you've already read enough about mine.

What about yours? What about those in your family? What issues aren't allowed to be discussed or accepted in our culture? In our businesses, schools, cities, homes?

We can face the issues, make wise decisions, and swim on the waters of a sea of hope. We can delete the mental music of denial and hate and bitterness and selfishness, letting songs of joy and endurance and wisdom and service now control our mental playlists.

My friend Justin Zuccarelli found a way:

> A little over seventeen years ago, I had my first tonic-clonic seizure. My life changed completely on November 3, 1999. It was half a lifetime ago. That day put me on a path I

never envisioned, but now I couldn't imagine things turning out any differently. I remember the fear, the anger, the stress, the confusion, and countless other emotions when I learned that I had had a seizure. The life I knew was made different by something out of my control. It was especially difficult because the first neurologist said he couldn't say I had epilepsy; he said I had a seizure disorder (I didn't know these are the same thing). About a year later, when a different neurologist told me I did have epilepsy, my perspective changed. For many people, a diagnosis such as this is devastating, but for me, it was a relief. My seizures didn't necessarily affect me negatively in specific ways (work, friendships, school, etc.), but it was like a cloud over my life—always there, always on my mind. Now, this cloud had a name: epilepsy.

Living with epilepsy has become my new normal. Even though I am seizure free, the cloud is still there; however, the light shines through more often than not. Epilepsy and other invisible disorders, diseases, and disabilities have ruined many people's lives, but I am one of the lucky ones. Epilepsy has made me who I am. In spite of the adversity I've faced because of my seizures, I wouldn't trade having epilepsy because of the incredible people and opportunities I've had as a result. I have been able to move past my diagnosis and work to help others by advocating for them, by sharing my experiences, and by helping others so they are able to manage their epilepsy.

This quotation from William Shakespeare's Julius Caesar (Act I; Scene 2; 249–260) is relevant to my adventure underwater:

Casca: He fell down in the market place and foamed at mouth and was speechless.

Brutus: 'Tis very like. He hath the falling sickness.

"Falling sickness" was a term once used for epilepsy. The first tonic-clonic seizure I had on that day in 1999 was when I was wearing a shirt from the band Falling Sickness. That eerie coincidence will always give me chills.

Or like my friend, Nathan Jirovec, who lives with epilepsy but carries the weight of his brother's death in a car accident—though his own damage was so severe, the family thought he was the one who died. He writes about his story, about watching a video of his own funeral, about the questions of why he lived and his brother didn't. He can swim.

Matysan Harper felt "swallowed by the ocean that day," she said. "Not being in control over my own life was suffocatingly surreal. I didn't have a choice but to trust God. That surrender meant getting new breath in my lungs, and a new life that I didn't have to worry about figuring out on my own." When she sings, those in the audience also feel a new life at sea. "Singing, and music in general, helps me feel peace," she says. "My story is much more than just that season of my life. That was not the end of my life song, although it very well could have been. I sing because I know that music gives voice to things beyond what I see underwater." She sings while swimming.

What's Helped Me

• Play a sport. For fun and growth, not stressful competition. And remember your limitations.

Chris Maxwell

Like my friend, Amy Wyatt, who tells amazing stories about her son and his life with epilepsy. Through determination, prayer, and the pursuit of the best options possible, Amy smiles hearing her son tell his own story. They can swim.

Like hearing my friend Phil Gattone tell his story about life with epilepsy. He found ways to endure the swift currents, to adjust to cruel waves, and to stare defeat in the face. He's chosen to become part of the larger epilepsy tribe, embracing our diversity and acknowledging our need for community. He can swim, and through his hard work and great mind on technology, he is helping us all swim better. Phil tells us: "Never settle. Keep looking for a way to live better. Don't let anyone tell you what you can't do. Set your own standards and goals, and put everything you've got into meeting them."

Like a soldier coming back from war with traumatic brain injury, like the woman whose own family refuses to visit her because of their odd view about epilepsy, like the caregiver who knows that love hurts but refuses to either deny or control. We can all swim.

And we swim best when choosing to live life correctly.

So find the spoons, and keep them close. Open your eyes, and see the wonder underwater. Choose to welcome the life around you. Fall in love with your own ocean—remember to see the depths beyond the visual limitations. Assist anyone struggling to swim nearby—remember this ocean of existence includes everyone with a battle.

I recently processed all this again as my sister and brother-in-law allowed me to drive their boat on Lake Hartwell. Debbie sat near the back with Janet, while Bruce calmly stood near me in my role as operator. Glancing at a shining sun and a bright blue sky, hearing the rhythm of waves and the power of a boat, feeling the motion, listening to Debbie and Janet talk though not able to hear their words, I breathed. Calmly enjoying the moment. Remembering Mama and oceans and baby boys and meals and mornings and evenings, while riding on the water of then—a time of awe, a segment of trust, a reflection of endurance. I wasn't sure what they were thinking, but I was contemplating my thinking.

I steered toward a shore. We turned off the engine and rested. Listening to some songs reminding us about life, swimming in water we had no control over, laughing a few times, we saw the wonder. And as my mind thought thoughts none of them knew, a little moisture came from my eyes—like tiny waves of healing from a deep sea housing two decades of wounds.

Then and there, I gained a healthy glance of this life underwater.

I want us all to gain that.

Because the adventure underwater is beautiful.

The adventure underwater is frightening.

What's Helped Me

- Drive—or if you aren't able to drive, ask your driver to drive—a different route home. Refuse to always take the same roads at the same time. (This one is very hard for me. Not only because am I a man of habit, but it also helps me not forget. Still, I have learned a few new turns bring me a fresh look and also help my brain. Give it a try.).

Chris Maxwell

The adventure underwater is dangerous.

The adventure underwater requires preparation.

The adventure underwater is impossible to fully prepare for.

The adventure underwater reveals realities never known on the shore.

Remember. And choose today to relax. Reflect on your time spent at sea. Realize you are called for a retreat, a rest, a recovery.

Swim ashore.

Dry off, slowly.

Walk into the nearby restaurant, slowly.

Place an order, even if you struggle to remember.

Receive your meal.

Sit.

Eat, slowly.

Enjoy.

This is your time.

Conclusion: The Shore

I am trying to become a living human being. I am trying to know more fully how to love, grieve, sing, befriend, forgive, heal, and give thanks. So often suffering gets in the way. I wish it were not so, yet all of us inevitably must pass through the shadowlands of doubt and despair. I wish it were not so. But it is so. None of us are exempt. There is only trusting and seeking and failing and then trusting again.[56] —Mark Yaconelli

And faith is, in the end, a kind of homesickness—for a home we have never visited but have never once stopped longing for.[57] —Philip Yancey

The night's presentation declared wonder—a clear spring sky exposing the beauty of stars smiling. Clouds departed. Darkness appearing friendly, my mind imagined my own constellations. A wide world imparted images for an imagination to see in its way, its time, its method.

No longer concealed. Revealed.

No longer hidden. Exposed.

Sensation invited, at least inside me. While alone. While thinking. While dreaming. While imagining. Perceiving fictional pictures stimulated by nonfictional characters far away but near on that night, in my mind, with me.

Should we call it dreaming? Thinking? Imagining? Should we call it exercising the mental system?

Systems keep us stable. They guide, direct, lure, inspire. They protect and provide. They can also become damaged, causing malfunctions in unexpected times. They can overreact, causing ongoing storms amid the constellations of normality.

Brains can be systems fitting all those categories. My brain is. My brain does.

---

56 *The Gift of Hard Things*, 143.
57 *Disappointment with God*, 246.

The mental electrical system—hidden by a bald head and a skull, masked by prepared agenda and rehearsed smiles, covered by sincere care and bare confessions—can feel like a clear sky on a calm night. But it can change. It does change. It becomes—sometimes slowly, sometimes suddenly—a storm. Winds rage. Thunder hits the stage and gets all the attention. Lightning strikes.

From image to reality, what does that mean? When the brain struggles because of scar tissue, learning and remembering and communicating labor to do their assigned duties. Maybe slowly, feeling tired and weak and dizzy. Maybe suddenly, scrambling to stutter a word.

A creative sentence written. An inspiring phrase stated. Then? A name forgotten, a nap needed, a mood shifting, an emotion appearing like a cloud barging in to redesign a sky's beauty on a lovely evening in Georgia.

Though it has issues, I try hard to work well with this mind of mine. I know her weaknesses, her tendencies, her barriers. She strives to overcompensate for her scars. The obsession with work overworks her as she seeks to locate words hidden deep inside her damaged region.

But my mind moved away from herself and dwelled again on the marvel above. For then, she just gazed at the sky's grace. She needed a moment, gazing at a sky smiling down, telling her and telling me to rest, to be still, to just be.

That is how I feel coming ashore. Leaving, for a moment, the waves of epilepsy.

I remember, though, that those around me need their own shores.

I mentioned Taylor and Aaron in the book. Graham, our youngest son and a basketball coach, also offered his own thoughts. They fit here, as we near this adventure's end:

> I am probably the lucky one out of all of our close family. I was so young I do not exactly remember how my dad was before his illness. I just know he changed. I just know he struggled with things he didn't struggle with before. But I also saw resilience in him and my mom. Both of them are fighters.
>
> Most people don't always remember an event or even a specific person. They remember how that event or person made them feel. I just remember how I felt during that time period. It was just confusion. Was I going to have a dad

anymore? Was my dad ever going to get better? Would his memory ever come back to him? I just had questions and there never seemed to be any answers.

But I found answers to questions I didn't even ask. What does love look like? It looks like my mom loving my dad through such difficult times when most people would've hung it up. It looks like my brothers taking care of me and shielding me from the reality no seven-year-old should see. What is forgiveness? It looks like forgiving yourself before you can forgive others. It looks like forgiving others even when they don't ask for it.

My dad became a new person after his illness. Our whole family felt underwater for several years. But when you can finally come up for air and see sky and the birds, you learn to appreciate the moments that forced you to fight and swim. We are all swimming in our ways in life. But that certain experience with my dad has forced me to become a better swimmer, even when I didn't ask for it. For that, I am thankful.

What ways are you swimming? How do you adjust to live with questions when you see no answers beside them? Have you learned to appreciate the moments? What should you do to help yourself and others find hope at sea and peace at the shore?

Well, a recent encounter reminded me of the bigger issues of life underwater. This story, I believe, will be a nice conclusion—or maybe an invitation to a new adventure on the water.

My latest EEG was scheduled for early one Monday morning, so I spent Sunday night in Atlanta. After meeting with a friend, I took time in the hotel room to rest and read and write—three key life goals for me. Then I remembered it was time to take my anti-epileptic meds and time to eat. To me, that is time for a major decision. I wanted a place nearby and inexpensive.

I remembered McDonalds had started serving breakfast all day. I searched my phone for the nearest one. That caused another problem—I had three selections to choose from. Those who know me would expect me to choose to closest. For an odd reason, I decided to select the one in the middle.

I grabbed my meds and let my phone steer me to dinner. The location didn't look like the safest, so I briefly questioned my major life decision—did I choose the right McDonalds?

Too late to change. It was time for dinner breakfast and meds. I parked and walked in, facing another decision. Would I eat in or get it to go so I could get work done at the hotel while eating?

I stayed in. I needed a break, a rest, a few moments to eat in a place I had never been before. I needed to come ashore and deal with my thoughts about the next morning's EEG.

I began eating by the window.

And then I saw people coming toward McDonalds. Many people. Walking. Adults—not wearing nice clothes but looking very hungry.

They entered, loudly.

Two—a man and a woman—walked near my table. The man slammed a trash bag of stuff at a table across from me.

"I'm here by myself," I said. "I can move to a smaller table if you guys are a group needing room to eat together."

"No," he mumbled. "We're fine."

He talked to the lady I assumed to be his wife. He told her what he wanted for dinner. She went to place an order, standing in the long line of men and women of various colors and ages.

The man then sat at the table across from me.

I repeated my previous statement, wanting him to know I could move if that was best.

"No," he said again. "If I ever get to eat at McDonalds, I want to sit right here."

His face and his voice indicated there was so much more to his story. I wanted to know his story. I wanted to know about his own life underwater.

I asked him to tell me his story.

And he did.

He told me of his previous career, of raising a family, of economic problems, of now living with his wife on the streets of Atlanta.

A man and his wife in a big city. A family. A former solid vocation. No home. No money to afford their own food. One trash bag carrying all their possessions.

I asked more questions. He told me more of his story—not asking for anything in return, just telling me his life underwater.

I finished my dinner breakfast and asked, "Who brought all of you here to eat?" He pointed near the counter, showing me the man.

I wanted to meet that man. I wanted to be like him if I ever grow up.

Before walking out in my casual shoes and getting in my comfortable car and driving to a hotel and sleeping inside instead of the streets and preparing for a morning EEG, I met Scott Smith.

What does love look like?

That night I saw what love looks like.

Love looks like Scott bringing many homeless people to McDonalds for dinner.

Scott was as kind as I was nosey. I wanted to know what inspired a man to purchase meals for the homeless. He answered with words, but also with his heart.

And he wanted to know about me.

Scott displayed a desire to rescue a world of those living underwater. One life at a time. One meal at a time. One Sunday evening near Atlanta at a time.

I felt like I had just learned one of the biggest life lessons of how I should deal with my own scars—care for the scars of others.

Scott taught me that.

I drove slowly to my hotel and slept well. I woke early, wrote, read some assignments from my students, ate breakfast, and drove to have my brain checked.

Someone called as I drove, but I couldn't answer. My phone was guiding me toward my destination.

I arrived, as always, early. Before entering my EEG encounter, I called the number not knowing who it was.

"I received a call from this number."

"Hey, Chris, this is Scott," he said. "I met you last night at McDonalds. I asked why you were in town, and you told me you had some medical tests this morning. I just wanted you to know I am praying for you."

What does love look like?

That is what it looks like.

We had talked only once. But he called. He called to see if I was okay underwater.

I want the heart of Scott to guide me toward my destination. Underwater, brain damaged, living with epilepsy, I want to go there with that heart no matter what my head is like.

Content, unashamed, and courageous, I want to go there. To that place I belong. As me, a man who suffered from encephalitis, who lives with mental weaknesses, who lives with epilepsy, I want to go there. A place of love and care, of stories, of breakfast for dinner, of listening, of making a call to ask how someone is doing, of serving those who have no way to serve themselves.

Don't you?

Let's go there.

I hope we can meet underwater, smiling at the wonder nearby.

What does love look like?

Just maybe, love looks like us—those who know about life underwater.

Glossary

absence seizures: An absence seizure causes a short period of "blanking out" or staring into space.

Automated External Defibrillator (AED): a portable device that checks the heart rhythm and can send an electric shock to the heart to try to restore a normal rhythm. AEDs are used to treat sudden cardiac arrest (SCA). SCA is a condition in which the heart suddenly and unexpectedly stops beating.

Alzheimer's: *Alzheimer's is a type of dementia that causes problems with memory, thinking and behavior.* Symptoms usually develop slowly and get worse over time, becoming severe enough to interfere with daily tasks.

Auras: a type of simple focal seizure that becomes a generalized seizure (see secondarily generalized seizure). Auras are usually strange sensations, such as a strange smell, funny taste, or strange 'rising' feeling in the stomach. The person will be conscious and aware that the aura is happening. Auras are also sometimes called 'warnings' because they warn the person that a generalized seizure is coming.

complex partial seizures: These seizures usually start in a small area of the temporal lobe or frontal lobe of the brain. They quickly involve other areas of the brain that affect alertness and awareness. So even though the person's eyes are open and they may make movements that seem to have a purpose, in reality "nobody's home." If the symptoms are subtle, other people may think the person is just daydreaming.

Dementia: *Dementia is not a specific disease. It's an overall term that describes a wide range of symptoms* associated with a decline in memory or other thinking skills severe enough to reduce a person's ability to perform everyday activities.

Encephalitis: an inflammation of the brain caused by a virus. The major risk is permanent brain damage.

febrile seizures: Children aged 3 months to 5 or 6 years may have tonic-clonic seizures when they have a high fever. These are called febrile seizures (pronounced FEB-rile) and occur in 2 percent to 5 percent of all children. There is a slight tendency for them to run in families. If a child's parents, brothers or sisters, or other close relatives have had febrile seizures, the child is a bit more likely to have them.

generalized seizures: seizures that happen in, and affect, both sides of the brain from the start. There are many different types of generalized seizures but they all involve the person becoming unconscious, even just for a few seconds, and they won't remember the seizure itself. The most well-known generalized seizure is the tonic-colonic (convulsive) seizure.

Gustatory aura: characterized by taste phenomena including acidic, bitter, salty, sweet, or metallic tastes. Gustatory aura occur in seizures involving the parietal operculum and the insula.

herpes simplex virus encephalitis (HSVE): Herpes simplex encephalitis is a rare neurological condition that is characterized by inflammation of the brain (encephalitis). People affected by this condition may experience a headache and fever for up to five days, followed by personality and behavioral changes; seizures; hallucinations; and altered levels of consciousness. Without early diagnosis and treatment, severe brain damage or even death may occur. Herpes simplex encephalitis is caused by a virus called the herpes simplex virus.

Juvenile Myoclonic Epilepsy or JME: a form of epilepsy that starts in childhood or adolescence. People with this disorder experience muscle twitching or jerking. They may also have other seizure types, including full-blown convulsive seizures or absence seizures (staring spells).

MRI or **Magnetic Resonance Imaging**: Magnetic resonance imaging *(MRI)* is a test that uses a magnetic field and pulses of radio wave energy to make pictures of organs and structures inside the body. In many cases, *MRI* gives different information about structures in the body than can be seen with an X-ray, ultrasound, or computed tomography (CT) scan.

myoclonic seizures: Myoclonic seizures are brief shock-like jerks of a muscle or group of muscles. They occur in a variety of epilepsy syndromes that have different characteristics. During a myoclonic seizure, the person is usually awake and able to think clearly.

Olfactory aura: characterized by olfactory phenomena - usually an odor, which is often unpleasant. Olfactory aura occur in seizures involving the mesial temporal or orbitofrontal regions.

PET Scan: A positron emission tomography (PET) scan is an imaging test that allows doctors to check for disease in your body. The scan uses radioactive tracers in a special dye. These tracers are injected into a vein in your arm and are then absorbed by your organs and tissues.

post-traumatic seizure: are seizures that result from traumatic brain injury (TBI), brain damage caused by physical trauma. PTS may be a risk factor for post-traumatic epilepsy (PTE), but a person who has a seizure or seizures due to traumatic brain injury does not necessarily have PTE, which is a form of epilepsy, a chronic condition in which seizures occur repeatedly.

PTSD (post-traumatic stress disorder): a mental health problem that some people develop after experiencing or witnessing a life-threatening event, like combat, a natural disaster, a car accident, or sexual assault.

Seizure: A seizure is a sudden surge of electrical activity in the brain. It usually affects how a person appears or acts for a short time. Many different things can occur during a seizure. Whatever the brain and body can do normally can also occur during a seizure. Seizures are not a disease in themselves. Instead, they are a symptom of many different disorders that can affect the brain. Some seizures can hardly be noticed, while others are totally disabling.

Simple partial seizures: can be motor seizures that cause change in muscle activity, sensory seizures that cause changes in any one of the senses, autonomic seizures that cause changes in the part of the nervous system that automatically controls bodily functions, or psychic seizures that change how people think, feel, or experience things.

SUDEP: the sudden, unexpected death of someone with epilepsy

Traumatic brain injury (TBI): an intracranial injury, is generally the result of a sudden, violent blow or jolt to the head. The brain is launched into a collision course with the inside of the skull, resulting in possible bruising of the brain, tearing of nerve fibers and bleeding.

temporal lobe seizures: Temporal lobe seizures originate in the temporal lobes of your brain, which process emotions and are important for short-term memory. Some symptoms of a temporal lobe seizure may be related to these functions, including having odd feelings — such as euphoria, deja vu or fear.

to seize: to have a seizure

tonic-clonic seizures: The tonic-clonic seizure is what most people think of when they think of a convulsive seizure. A person loses consciousness, muscles stiffen, and jerking movements are seen. These types of seizures usually last 1 to 3 minutes and take much longer for a person to recover. A tonic-clonic seizure lasting more than 5 minutes is a medical emergency.

V-fib (ventricular fibrillation): a heart rhythm problem that occurs when the heart beats with rapid, erratic electrical impulses. This causes pumping chambers in your heart (the ventricles) to quiver uselessly, instead of pumping blood.

Vagal Nerve Stimulator or VNS: Vagus nerve stimulation (VNS Therapy®) is designed to prevent seizures by sending regular, mild pulses of electrical energy to the brain via the vagus nerve. These pulses are supplied by a device something like a pacemaker. The VNS device is sometimes referred to as a "pacemaker for the brain."

Wada Test: WADA testing is a procedure performed during angiography that assesses which side of your brain has your language and memory functions. During the test, one side of the brain is put to sleep (anesthetized) by injecting a medication into the carotid artery.

Sources

http://www.epilepsy.com/

https://www.epilepsysociety.org.uk/

http://www.alz.org/

www.webmd.com/

https://rarediseases.info.nih.gov/

www.mayoclinic.org/

Web sites/Resources

For further information, contact:

www.epilepsy.com

www.epilepsyadvocate.com

The following article has helpful information and encouragement for caregivers:

https://www.psychologytoday.com/blog/professor-cromer-learns-read/201203/after-brain-injury-the-dark-side-personality-change-part-i

Debbie Hampton, *The Best Brain Possible.*

www.TheBestBrainPossible.com

http://blog.mangohealth.com

About Chris Maxwell

Chris Maxwell is a husband, father, and grandfather. He is a writer, spiritual life director, international speaker, and a man who loves people. Chris hopes to be a voice of encouragement through words spoken, words written, and a life lived—at times, underwater.

Website/Blog: www.chrismaxwell.me

Twitter: @CMaxMan

Facebook: Facebook.com/PausewithChrisMaxwell

Email: CMaxMan11@gmail.com

Other Books by Chris Maxwell

Beggars Can Be Chosen: An Inspirational Journey Through the Invitations of Jesus

Changing My Mind: A Journey of Disability and Joy

Unwrapping His Presence: What We Really Need for Christmas

Pause: The Secret to a Better Life, One Word at a Time

Pause for Moms: Finding Rest in a Too Busy World

Pause for Pastors: Finding Still Waters in the Storm of Ministry

Pause with Jesus: Encountering His Story in Everyday Life